DECOLONIZING MEDICINE

DECOLONIZING MEDICINE

*Indigenous Politics and
the Practice of Care in Bolivia*

GABRIELA ELISA MORALES

STANFORD UNIVERSITY PRESS
Stanford, California

Stanford University Press
Stanford, California

Printed in the United States of America

Library of Congress Cataloging-in-Publication Data
Names: Morales, Gabriela Elisa, author.
Title: Decolonizing medicine : Indigenous politics and the practice of care in Bolivia / Gabriela Elisa Morales.
Description: Stanford, California : Stanford University Press, 2025. | Includes bibliographical references and index.
Identifiers: LCCN 2024047837 (print) | LCCN 2024047838 (ebook) | ISBN 9781503640856 (cloth) | ISBN 9781503642720 (paperback) | ISBN 9781503642737 (epub)
Subjects: LCSH: Indians of South America—Medical care—Bolivia. | Medical policy—Bolivia. | Decolonization—Bolivia.
Classification: LCC RA461 .M67 2025 (print) | LCC RA461 (ebook) | DDC 362.10984—dc23/eng/20250203

LC record available at https://lccn.loc.gov/2024047837
LC ebook record available at https://lccn.loc.gov/2024047838

Cover design: Susan Zucker
Cover art: Syringe: Shutterstock / Andychi; Chamomile: iStock / Anya Kami; Coca: Shutterstock / Morphart Creation

For my parents, Jorge and Silvia

CONTENTS

FIGURES

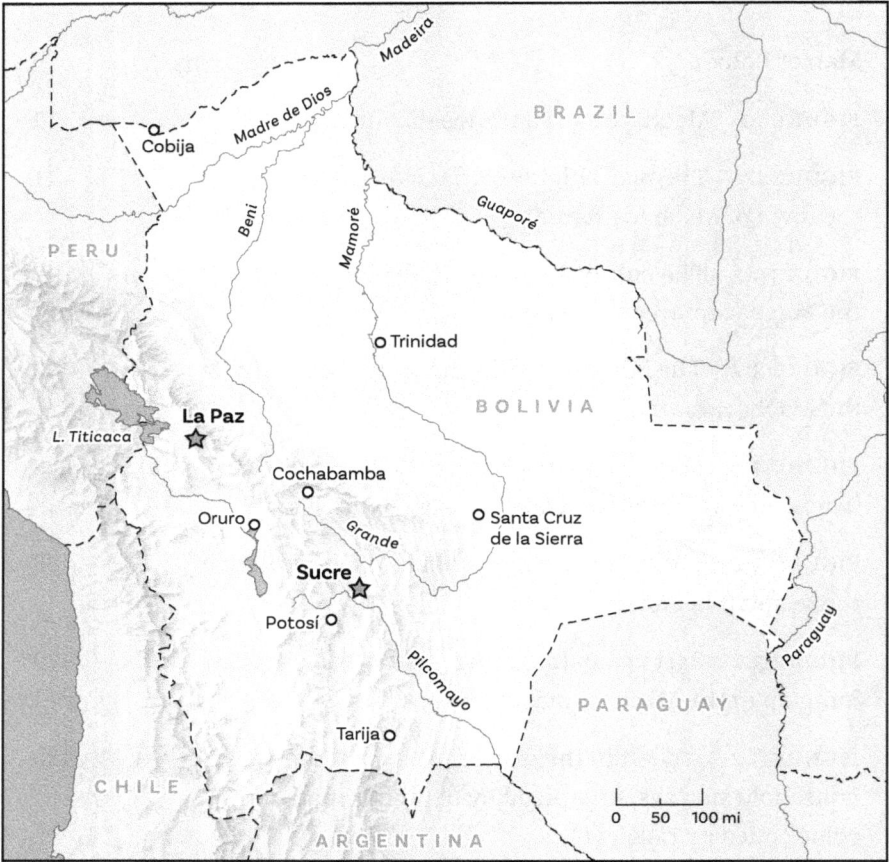

MAP 1. Map of Bolivia

It was July 2022—and everything had changed. I sat on a passenger plane circling ever lower through the thin atmosphere over the city of El Alto. With the outbreak of the Covid-19 pandemic, it had been three years since I was able to travel to see my extended family, friends, and research interlocutors in Bolivia. The sight of the growing sprawl of lights against the shadowed backdrop of mountains felt familiar, like coming home. And yet, nothing was the same.

The last time I had traveled to Bolivia was in July 2019 to wrap up research on a project on state-led efforts to decolonize the national health care system during the presidency of Evo Morales. Morales, first elected in 2005 and lauded as Bolivia's first Indigenous president, had undertaken what his administration described as a sweeping project to overturn colonial systems of oppression, including in areas such as health care. A few short months after that trip, in November 2019, President Morales was ousted from office—an event I followed from afar by reading news and social media coverage. The year that Morales's successor, the right-wing interim president Jeanine Añez, stayed in office had been difficult for many Bolivians. Her administration launched criminal investigations into members of the opposition and was responsible for two massacres that killed twenty-two protestors (Farthing and Becker 2021).

The political crisis worsened also with the onset of the Covid-19 pandemic in March 2020. The Añez administration initially enacted a strict lockdown. As I discuss in the Conclusion, these punitive approaches especially targeted and burdened rural Indigenous and *campesino* (peasant) communities. Despite early lockdown measures to mitigate contagion, uneven health infrastructures limited the availability of health services and key supplies like oxygen. Estimates suggested that if excess deaths in 2020 were counted, Bolivia had one of the highest death tolls from Covid in the world (Foronda and UDAPE 2023; Trigo, Kurmanaev, and McCann 2020).

By the time I landed in Bolivia again, both the political and health landscapes had shifted once more. New national elections were held in October 2020, and Luis Arce won the presidency. He was from Evo Morales's party—the Movement Toward Socialism (*Movimiento al Socialismo*, MAS)—and had promised to restore the progressive social and economic policies of the Morales era. By 2021, vaccines were becoming available in the Global North—but what some have termed global "vaccine apartheid" (Bajaj, Maki, and Stanford 2022) meant that countries in the Global South like Bolivia could not access them until much later. The Arce administration worked to cobble together vaccines from various sources, including the World Health Organization's COVAX program, Russia, and China. Even as global travel restrictions had started to loosen, I was hesitant to return to Bolivia before vaccines were widely and regularly available, as I did not want to potentially expose people who did not have access to protections from the virus. In July 2022, it seemed that things were finally looking up, as case numbers were going down and more and more people had gotten their second and third shots in the vaccine sequence. Even so, it was not smooth sailing: Bolivia, like many places, was still recovering from the devastation of the early pandemic years and dealing with the ongoing effects of new variant waves.

I completed much of the research for this book in Bolivia before Evo Morales's ouster and before the onset of the global Covid-19 pandemic.

But writing this book amid twinned political and health crises—what many in Bolivia called the "double pandemic"—prompted me to continually revisit my arguments and approach. The pandemic threw into sharp relief long-standing resource inequalities between Global North and Global South; and in many contexts around the world, structural inequalities made it so that the pandemic disproportionately affected low-income, racialized, and disabled populations. As national and global health policymakers sought to respond to the pandemic, solutions often fell short and reentrenched existing forms of inequity and structural violence. The need for imaginative policy alternatives—for substantive transformations that might better address structural inequities in health care—is ever more urgent.

But even as the need remains pressing, it is hard not to turn to pessimism. At its heart, this is a book about the contingencies and limitations of policy reform in a context of enduring colonialism. In part, this book follows how Bolivian officials under the Morales administration sought to radically reimagine health care services under a framework of *descolonización* (decolonization) that brought together Indigenous anticolonial projects, social medicine, and community health approaches. It also follows how, over the course of design and implementation, these projects unevenly folded back into liberal reformist paradigms that were also more in line with regional and global models of managing cultural difference within the health care system. In many instances, health interventions ended up reinscribing, rather than challenging, long-standing colonial modes of care. I argue such reinscriptions cannot simply be ascribed to state "failure" or even, as some would have it, state hypocrisy. Instead, they reflect a complex nexus of material and ideological flows. The turn to more limited policy approaches in part reflected infrastructural shortages and unequal global resource distribution that constrained policy action. At the same time, limitations also reflected how colonial, racializing, and gendered modes of categorization, intervention, and habituated care remained sticky and were continually reinvented amid explicitly stated projects to undo them.

At this same time, in grappling with critique, I also had to reckon with the existence of worse alternatives. The interim Añez administration gutted many Morales-era health programs—and its punitive pandemic response revealed how replicating racist narratives of contagion and failing to provide sufficient socioeconomic support to endure lockdowns intensified harm on multiple scales. Witnessing these shifts—albeit from afar—pushed me to ask hard questions of myself about the role of academic critique in understanding the workings of unequal systems. How might critique attend to substantial differences across administrations, as well as continuities in broader structures? At the same time, how might critique analyze enduring structures of settler colonialism across administrations while also not assuming that their replication is total or inevitable (Lambert 2022; Simpson 2014)?

In thinking through these questions, conversations with my interlocutors have pushed me to also see political possibilities in critique. Over the course of my research, countless patients, civil society leaders, practitioners, and others continually analyzed and critiqued the structural and political systems that shaped their encounters with health care. Frequently, patients and civil society leaders verbally articulated these critiques in the form of public-facing complaints—complaints that drew attention to enduring problems of unequal resource distribution and medical mistreatment. Paying attention to such moments points to how localized forms of critique beyond the academy can operate in ways that are closely tied to building new political futures. As political scientist Thea Riofrancos, writing about Indigenous environmental activist movements during Rafael Correa's presidency in Ecuador, reminds us, "Critique is a genre of discourse that endeavors to reveal the root causes and systemic nature of its object. . . . [T]he practice of critique also opens up the possibility of—and the demand for—a world otherwise" (2020, 17). For my interlocutors, complaints were often a means to reshuffle relationships with state and nonprofit institutions and hold them accountable to political promises; they also laid the groundwork for enacting worlds where more dignified living might be possible.

In writing this book, I ask what possibilities might be opened up when academic critique is guided by and responsive to quotidian, lo-

calized forms of critique. While recognizing the importance of analyzing systems of power, scholars have also increasingly debated the
shortcomings of academic critique. It can treat colonial systems as
totalizing (Lambert 2022), it can position the scholar as authoritative
"debunker" (Latour 2004), and it can also foreclose action (Ahmed
2006). Even as it analyzes power, critique can sometimes appear removed from social struggles. Foregrounding interlocutors' practices of
critique does not necessarily solve the tensions and complicities built
into academic writing. Like the policies I describe in this book, academic knowledge production is often bound up in the very systems that
authors may aspire to critique and undo—particularly given that books
like this one are written in English for a largely academic audience (although it will also be translated into Spanish). But such foregrounding
might be a step toward co-theorization—and toward engaging critique
as a generative, rather than a foreclosing, practice. Critique might in
itself be a form of demanding policy accountability amid deepening
inequality; it might offer a move toward building a more hopeful political future.

As I was growing up in the United States, my father sought to help me
maintain my connections to his home country from afar. My father,
originally from a middle-class *mestizo* family in Cochabamba, Bolivia,
had left the country when he was eighteen. He received a scholarship
to study at a university in Switzerland, where he met my mother, a
white woman from a working-class family in the rural Rhine Valley.
Our family moved from Switzerland to the States when I was four years
old. As I was growing up, my father would cook picante de pollo and
pastel de choclo for us. He told my brother and me stories about our
relatives and about the town of Cochabamba. He also told us jokes that
were humorous but had an undertone of seriousness—satirical sayings
about the Bolivian dictator Hugo Banzer, whose hard-fisted rule and
continual threats to shut down universities in the 1980s was one reason
my father left the country.

When I turned eighteen—the same age as my father was when he left Bolivia—we went on a trip to Bolivia together so that I could meet my extended family for the first time. A few months before, Evo Morales had just been inaugurated as president for his first term in office. With his election and inauguration still fresh, his proposed reforms were a source of active debate at the dinner tables and gatherings where I met my many aunts, uncles, and cousins. Despite our shared last name, our family was not related to the president. But most of my relatives followed politics and the news closely, and several of them had also worked for the national government at various points in time. My uncle Rolando, a socialist economist and university professor in La Paz, went to work for Evo Morales's administration for several years at the head of the office of business regulation. His son, my cousin Camilo, an industrial engineer, worked for the Vice-Ministry of Development for multiple terms. Other relatives, however, were less enthusiastic about Evo Morales's election. My uncle Juan Antonio, also an economics professor in La Paz, had been at the head of the Central Bank under the administration of neoliberal president Sánchez de Lozada in the 1990s; he identified as a liberal centrist and was highly critical of the Morales administration's approach. My aunt Beatriz, who had previously had to go into hiding after mobilizing against the dictatorship of Luis García Meza, frequently expressed her support for the MAS. My other aunt, Luly, considerably more conservative than all her siblings, vocally shared her disapproval. Politics, in short, was often a source of contention and debate, and a way our family came together.

After that first trip, I returned to Bolivia nearly every year and also lived there for longer stretches for work. Over the course of those visits, and as I followed national politics, I also solidified my own political views, as well as a growing interest in the workings of the state. As a Bolivian citizen, I voted for Evo Morales's reelection—yet my understanding of the MAS was also increasingly accompanied by a sense of the party's contradictions and limitations. The 2012 march of Tsimané, Yuracaré, and Mojeño-Trinitario protesters against the Morales administration's proposed construction of a highway through their protected territory was a turning point in national conversations;

the widely covered protest brought to the fore tensions between the state's promise of decolonization and its ongoing reliance on extractive development in the oil- and gas-rich lowlands. Beyond these highly visible protests, other social movements that once supported the MAS increasingly criticized it for backtracking on some of its promises. Even as I continued to support the MAS in elections (seeing it as far better than the other options), I grappled with its contradictions—with how the party had brought concrete progressive changes while also encountering limitations and reproduced state systems of violence and extraction.

My concern with the conditions and limitations of political transformation also began to converge with a growing interest in health care, particularly as I moved through various standpoints within health care systems in both Bolivia and the United States. Over the years, I worked in the field of public health, cared for sick relatives in hospital settings, and also navigated care as a patient with chronic pain. These varied experiences turned my attention to another set of contradictions: when efforts to provide for others might be inadequate to addressing the unequal structures shaping people's lives, or when these efforts might even generate new forms of exclusion. For example, when I worked for a year as a research assistant on a dengue fever prevention project for the National Center for Tropical Diseases in Santa Cruz, Bolivia, people frequently complained to us that they were being asked to throw out standing water they needed for chores. They pointed out that the municipal government itself had done little to address standing water accumulated in the streets. It was a contradiction that those of us on the team very much acknowledged—and yet it was easy to feel stymied as minor bureaucratic actors with little say over municipal or national government policies.

I came to these questions through a different route as I sought biomedical treatment for my chronic pain in the United States and partially in Bolivia. In medical encounters, practitioners' desires to help and care for me were often bound up in the assumptions they made about gender and disability. In a terrain of diagnostic uncertainty, some doctors assured me it was all in my head or asked me if I could just try resuming normal activities. And yet, I am grateful too, for those doctors who did eventually find a diagnosis, those who sought to work with me to figure out treatment regimens with the acknowledgment that all care was piecemeal, that there might not be a cure. These varied medical encounters reminded me continually that medicine could be a site both of desire and of anxiety, of help and of harm.

I came to this research project because I wanted to learn from and engage with what it might mean to build a decolonized health care system and radically envision a different way of doing care. As I was doing this work, however, I also increasingly noticed resonant tensions between help and harm taking shape. Patients and practitioners I interviewed shared their desires for a biomedicine that would work for them—one that, very often, reflected the promises of a more dignified life promised by the Morales administration. At the same time, clinical and public health encounters often ended up being a place of further exclusion, where resource inequalities intersected with entrenched race, class, and gender hierarchies. I heard echoes of dynamics I had encountered before as a public health care worker, patient, and caregiver—even as the experiences I was talking to people about were structurally different from my own. I was working across key lines of difference, particularly as a non-Indigenous scholar doing research that centrally engaged with Indigenous anticolonial projects and the experiences of Indigenous healers and patients. The critiques developed by my interlocutors pulled my attention in new directions and urged me to think about both the possibilities and the limits of moves to care.

———

Cultural anthropology has long moved away from the idea that the researcher is a "fly on the wall" or objective observer of social practices; instead, we acknowledge the partiality of knowledge, as well as the ways one's positionality can shape how we ask questions, access spaces, and develop relationships with our interlocutors. Métis STS scholar Max Liboiron reminds readers that positioning is also a matter of ethical obligation, one that provides a means to

> understand where authors are speaking from, what ground they stand on, whom their obligations are to, what forms of sovereignty are being leveraged, what structures of privilege the settler state affords, and how we are related so that our obligations to one another as speaker and listener, writer and audience, can be specific enough to enact obligations to one another. . . . How has colonialism affected us differently? Introducing yourself is part of ethics and obligation, not punishment. (2021, 4)

These conversations have helped me think through the multiple layers of relation I have to place, as well as how I move through research spaces and participate in forms of obligation and accountability. Thinking on these questions challenges predominating notions that being from a place makes one an "insider researcher"—and instead asks us to attend to the conditions and hierarchies that continually shape our work (Chatterjee 2001). Here, too, I think about how my family has been tied to state processes. However indirectly, people I interviewed were also affected by the national economic and development policies that relatives worked on—whether that was an earlier generation of neoliberal policies or a more recent set of MAS policies. As I write about health policy implementation, I think about how I am always already entangled in the processes I am analyzing. Other entanglements come, too, from the wider ways that projects of colonization and nation-building, as well as globally unequal resource flows, continually structure my position within this project. When I note that the Bolivian side of my family largely identifies as mestizo, for example, this situates my extended family within a deeper history of national projects of *mestizaje* as assimilation and social whitening in Bolivia and elsewhere in Latin America; to be mestizo—particularly when tied to middle- and upper-class socioeconomic status—is also a form of being unmarked, to not experience the same kinds of discrimination that low-income Indigenous and campesino groups do (de la Cadena 2000; Macusaya

Cruz 2020; Molina 2021). In my case, being half-Bolivian and growing up abroad also centrally shaped how I did this work. I move through the world as a white cisgender woman, and in Bolivia, I often also get read as *gringa* (foreigner from the United States or Europe) because of my lightly accented Spanish, the ease of global movement offered by my U.S. passport, and my affiliation with a U.S. university.

Writing about these entanglements does not mean resolving them—instead, it is a means of engaging the messy contingencies and conditions that shape research, while also opening up room for discussion, reflection, and continual revisiting of methods. It is a way of working through how, in a book analyzing the workings of colonial and state structures, academic knowledge production does not escape these structures.

A key part of this work means thinking through how these conditions set the groundwork for how I was able to do this research and access spaces. For example, within institutional policymaking spaces—such as state and NGO offices—I was often welcomed as someone with the social capital and credentials of a foreign researcher, who might also either give an international platform to the work the Morales administration was doing or offer a reflection on what was and was not working with policy implementation. These connections also shaped how I came to base much of my research in the local public hospital of a highland municipality I anonymize as "Machacamarca." Policymakers and NGO staffers based in La Paz described it as an exemplar of state decolonial health policy reforms. That is, while they acknowledged that policy implementation was very much a work-in-progress, they held up the hospital as a place where intercultural health programing was fairly well established, in part because of decades of NGO work at the institution. NGO staffers introduced me to the hospital director, who granted me permission to site my research there. Hospital administrators and biomedical practitioners took the time to do interviews with me and allowed me to observe their work. In turn, they frequently expressed hopes I could draw attention to the challenges of their work; they often used the interviews to share their experiences but also discuss grievances.

While they shaped my early interest in Bolivian politics, my ex-tended family had little direct bearing on my research. I conducted my research independently of them, instead working to build connec-tions, initially through the NGO I shadowed, and later through word-of-mouth from interlocutors I had already interviewed. My relatives were not situated enough in the health care world that their names would have been widely recognized or gotten me access, nor did the power they held operate in a way that could have had consequences for my interlocutors. Put differently, they were public functionaries who had over time worked in different areas of government, but who had no sway over health care policy or health care resource distribution.

While I was able to interview policy and health actors and gain access to institutional spaces through these various modes of building relationships, I also had to attend to different concerns when seeking to build ethical relationships with patients, traditional healers and midwives, and others who often experienced these very institutions as sites of marginalization, ambivalence, and even violence. When working in Machacamarca, my race and educational and class status facilitated my ability to move through institutional spaces in a way that many of my interlocutors—who frequently experienced uncertainty and discrimination—could not. For example, in Chapter 3, I describe how biomedical practitioners granted me permission to sit in on child-births in the hospital, even as they frequently barred husbands and other family members of the patient for ostensibly disrupting biomed-ical work.

Other questions of obligation and accountability emerged in these moments, too. Patients, who had also granted me permission to be present, frequently positioned me as someone who could draw at-tention to their concerns and complaints about health care services. Like practitioners, they expressed frustrations about the limitations of health policy reform—but directed their concerns differently. They often emphasized experiences of neglect, mistreatment, and uncer-tainty as they navigated medical care.

Learning from the various kinds of critiques patients, practitioners, and other interlocutors developed—as well as their expectations that I might convey these critiques—has helped me to develop my analysis in this book. Being responsive to interlocutors' knowledge practices and ethical expectations is one way that I have sought to be accountable to my interlocutors. However, doing so also raised thorny questions about how to engage interlocutors' perspectives that were competing or coming from different standpoints. For example, patients I interviewed sometimes criticized biomedical practitioners for inadequate care, while biomedical practitioners sometimes shifted blame back onto patients. I sought to handle such moments by both attending to the directionality of power and locating practices within wider structures of material and social inequality. For instance, I have sought to foreground how biomedical practitioners can themselves be subject to race and class hierarchies, even as they also turn these onto patients within an entrenched system of colonial care. Ultimately, while I seek to represent all of my interlocutors as three-dimensional persons navigating complex systems, I prioritize the critiques put forward by my Aymara interlocutors who were trying to move through the health care system: patients, their family members, as well as healers and midwives whose uncompensated labor was being tangentially brought into the formal health care system.

But writing that foregrounds localized forms of critique is only one partial, imperfect mode of accountability among several. There were many ways that my interlocutors across various sites asked for accountability—for example, by suggesting approaches I might use for my project, asking I share findings with them, and requesting my participation in adjacent projects, like helping to write up an oral history of Machacamarca. As I describe in Chapter 5, a few families also invited me into kinship ties, following the forms of obligation that also took shape with institutional actors and others in positions of relative power. The work of accountability is ongoing and does not end with what is written on the page.

Critique, as I came to understand it in conversation with people I interviewed, was one means to hold others in positions of relative power—including state officials, biomedical practitioners, and researchers like me—accountable. Many of my interlocutors who were patients and residents of Machacamarca had voted for Evo Morales and were supporters of the MAS. At the same time, they actively critiqued health policies and other state programs that were falling short of promised changes; for many, the MAS, while offering an important step forward, did not always go far enough in its enactments of decolonization and material redistribution. My interlocutors also actively critiqued practitioners' care in the hospital. They also on occasion critiqued me and offered suggestions when they thought I should do things differently. (For example, several interlocutors reminded me of the importance of returning to visit them and sharing my findings; others offered critical feedback and suggestions on the oral history of the town I helped to write). Such localized practices of critique were at once a lively analytical, ethical, and political practice that could reshuffle relations for the better.

While much of this book examines how efforts toward political transformation run up against challenges and reentrench longstanding structural inequalities, these reinscriptions are also not the end of the story. Building on the many conversations I had over the course of this research, I hope that this scholarly work of critique might align with demands for more just and dignified forms of care. If nothing else, I hope readers come away with a sense that in Bolivia, activist struggles are ongoing—that they pushed for the changes brought about by the MAS and continue to push for more. Amid ongoing political and health crises (in Bolivia and elsewhere), the work of transformation is already under way.

DECOLONIZING MEDICINE

INTRODUCTION
WAITING FOR REFORM

IN THE WAITING ROOM OF the municipal hospital of Machacamarca,[1] a small but growing town in the Bolivian highlands, a large red and yellow sign hung overhead, welcoming patients in both Spanish and Aymara. The brightly painted, polished sign hung over rows of black chairs near the reception desk, where patients lined up starting at the crack of dawn to get an appointment slip for the day. The walls of the waiting room had also been painted a warm, peachy yellow at the hospital director's instruction—because, he insisted, it would create a more welcoming space for the region's majority Indigenous Aymara residents, whom he described as preferring warmer colors.[2]

The bilingual sign and yellow walls were rarely a source of overt commentary among patients. Most, waiting for several hours for their name to be called after they received their appointment slips, chatted with other waiting patients. Some watched over their children, glee-fully running back and forth to pass the time, while other patients quietly stared up at the television on the far wall, which was usually showing reruns of *Los Simpsons* or *El Chavo del Ocho*.

As I was conducting ethnographic research in the hospital in 2015, I frequently chatted with patients in the waiting room who talked to me to pass the time, some sharing concerns about long trips from their home villages and long wait times ("es un quita tiempos"—"it's a waste of time"), others, uncertainties over whether doctors would be able to help. This was how, one morning, I met Violeta, a middle-aged woman whose son had broken his arm, and who was still waiting for the doctor to call them back in after her son had gotten an X ray that morning. Wryly glancing at those of us sitting nearby, she declared in a mix of Aymara and Spanish, "I bet the doctor doesn't even speak Aymara." As her small audience murmured in agreement, she looked around conspiratorially and, with laughter in her voice, said in Spanish, "Me va a decir, '¿Quéee?'" ("He will say, 'Whaaat?'"). She exaggerated the last syllable, parodying the tone that doctors sometimes used with patients.

The bilingual sign and yellow walls were among several additions to the hospital building undertaken in the name of creating an intercultural and decolonized space for the region's majority Indigenous Aymara residents. Although the original structure of the hospital closely mirrored the white-tiled, laboratory-like exam rooms long found in most public hospitals and clinics in Bolivia, later extensions to the building, funded by a transnational NGO, also added orange-hued birthing rooms and a greenhouse filled with medicinal plants. One of the existing exam rooms had also been given over to Aymara traditional healers so that they could care for patients in the hospital.

While a range of institutional actors—a transnational nonprofit organization, the municipal government, and the hospital director himself—made adjustments to the hospital architecture over the years, most were in agreement: the transformation of hospital space had largely been made possible by health care reforms under President Evo Morales Ayma. Governing from 2006 until his ouster in 2019, Bolivia's first Indigenous president undertook a sweeping series of reforms in the name of *descolonización* (decolonization), vowing to reverse intertwined colonial and capitalist systems of oppression and restore an Indigenous ethics of good living. Often, the decolonial project was rendered visible through material and symbolic markers in public institutions: the *wiphala*—the Indigenous social movement flag—flying over government buildings; the paintings of the Aymara revolutionary leaders, Túpac Katari and Bartolina Sisa, hanging in offices; a cable car public transport system in the nearby cities of La Paz and El Alto that likewise marked place names in both Aymara and Spanish. Hybrid efforts to transform the Machacamarca Hospital's built environment carried echoes of these other material projects and accumulated in seemingly warm spaces designed to make patients feel cared for.

Clinical architecture was one of several sites of care under the newly decolonized state, and it reflected broader policy transformations. In the realm of health care, policies invoking the framework of decolonization proposed the transformation of biomedical care practices to incorporate greater attentiveness and cultural competency, including by requiring practitioners to take Indigenous language classes appropriate to the region where they worked. They also included the incorporation of traditional healers and midwives into clinical settings, and greater community participation and decision making over local health policies.

Yet Violeta's offhand comment in the waiting room was not the first time I had been confronted with patients' criticisms (some of them humorous, some of them not) of clinical care. While the tenuousness of health care could be a subject of concern for many in Bolivia, it was especially so for low-income Indigenous patients, who often encountered long wait times and material shortages in public hospitals and clinics, as well as dynamics of paternalism, discrimination, and neglect. Even as various institutional energies had been put into reforming spaces and practices of care, many Aymara patients and residents of Machacamarca continued to describe their local hospital as a place *donde no hay atención* (a phrase that might be translated from Spanish as "where there is no treatment" or "where there is no care"). They continued to worry out loud about the violence and neglect they might encounter there.

Decolonizing Medicine is an ethnographic account of Bolivian state-led efforts to decolonize health care during Evo Morales's presidency—an account that shifts primarily between policymaking in the city of La Paz and care practices in the rural municipality I give the pseudonym of "Machacamarca." It emerges from a total of twenty-six months of ethnographic research I conducted in Bolivia between 2012 and 2019, with the longest continuous stretch unfolding over eighteen months from mid-2014 to the end of 2015. Engaging with the perspectives of patients, biomedical practitioners, traditional healers and midwives, community health representatives, NGO workers, and state bureaucrats, I consider how care becomes an ambivalent site of decolonial praxis. I demonstrate how Bolivian state and medical institutions turned to what I call *warm care* as the primary path to decolonial transformation; yet this focus on warm care unevenly reentrenched colonial moral paradigms. This reentrenchment had myriad material effects on relations, the body, and politics.

By "warm care," I refer to a cluster of moral, material, and affective care practices centered on a project of inclusivity, cultural sensitivity, and generally humane forms of attention. Sometimes, warm care was infused in signs and walls, accreted in peach-yellow paint and Aymara words of welcome. Other times, it permeated bodily gestures and ways of speaking and seeing. I argue that warm care became central to state efforts to decolonize health care in Bolivia by yoking an ongoing liberal paradigm of inclusion to the image of the newly caring state and its project of limited economic redistribution. I draw the term "warm care" from the common framing that practitioners were learning to provide care *con calidad y calidez* ("with quality and warmth")—a phrase also used elsewhere in Latin America.[3] In the Bolivian context, it was discursively bound up with state promises during Evo Morales's presidency to repair colonial-capitalist violence and restore Indigenous good living. This emergent mode of care created points of commensuration between multiple political goals of the Morales administration—and yet it also displaced other proposals for decolonization that came from activists and also, at times, from others working within the state apparatus.

ENDURING COLONIALISM

In tracing what Brian Johnson (2010) aptly calls the "paradoxes of decol-onization" in Bolivian health care, I approach biomedicine and public health as sites of enduring—if uneven and incomplete—colonialism. Numerous anthropological works have examined social inequality in Latin American health care systems, highlighting dynamics of racism, sexism, and classism as they play out across clinical encounters and modes of intervening in patient bodies. Medical anthropologists have especially emphasized how projects of neoliberal privatization and structural adjustment deepen health inequities and limit access to care.[4] At the same time, even while centering key processes of social stratification within health care systems, many analyses relegate dis-cussions of colonialism to a historical chapter—one that might have lingering influences on contemporary social formations but that is largely over. In doing so, discussions of health inequity risk replicating what Chickasaw anthropologist Shannon Speed describes as "the basic premise that the settler has settled, and is now from here, rather than acknowledging that there is a state of ongoing occupation, in Latin America as elsewhere in the hemisphere" (2017, 786).

In the rural but urbanizing town of Machacamarca, residents reck-oned with how colonialism was not an event in the past but continued to shape the present and spur illness. Located on either side of a major highway, the town had grown rapidly in recent years, as Aymara mi-grants from nearby villages left behind a life of agriculture or mining and moved to town to work in informal commerce and transport. Still, Aymara residents whose families had lived in Machacamarca for generations had long memories. In conversations with me, neigh-bors frequently invoked the site near the river where a Spanish colo-nial refining mill once stood. At night, mysterious fires burned and strange figures that appeared human but were not wandered about. If one stumbled across the site, one might go mad. Rumors about the haunted refining mill pointed to the enduring, illness-inducing effects of colonial and capitalist extraction.[5] Simultaneously, conversations with my interlocutors urged me to think about colonialism as an iterative process, one that manifested not only in the ghosts of the past, but could be continually found in enduring modes of social inequality. Understanding health inequity as tied to enduring colonialism points to the multifaceted ways that illness emerges from historical and ongoing projects of domination. Attending to these dynamics, moreover, foregrounds how medical institutions continually reinvent biopolitical regimes of intervening in racialized Indigenous patient bodies, replicating hierarchies of knowledge, and displacing local relations among human and other-than-human beings.

Indigenous movements and decolonial theorists across what are now known as the Americas have pointed to how, in contexts where European colonizers settled long term, colonialism did not end with formal independence from European crowns and the creation of new nation-states. When Indigenous movements across the hemisphere protest "five hundred years of colonialism," they point to the ways political, economic, ideological, and ontological orderings continue to maintain structures of domination over Indigenous communities and ongoing settler access to Indigenous land and labor.[6] As Aymara sociologist Silvia Rivera Cusicanqui has argued in her work on Bolivian history, "Both colonial transformations and those that emanated from liberal and populist reforms signified successive invasions and aggressions against Native peoples' and *ayllus'* forms of social, territorial, and economic and cultural organization. . . . [Reforms] introduced renewed mechanisms of oppression and material and cultural plunder" (2010, 41, my translation). Attending to these continuities across time does not entail collapsing past and present. Rather, it is a means of analyzing how projects of colonial domination are continually reinvented in new forms, including under projects of democratic and liberal state-building.

Particularly within Latin American contexts, scholars have emphasized how what Aníbal Quijano (1999; 2000) has called *la colonialidad del poder* (the coloniality of power) continues to operate through multiple scales and modes. They argue coloniality is a global system that has been co-constitutive with modernity and capitalism,[7] giving shape to Eurocentric epistemological and ontological hierarchies, material inequalities, and enduring formations of race, class, and gender.[8] Tracing the workings of coloniality in Latin America has on the one hand entailed looking toward global neocolonial knowledge production and economic resource flows, including those forged through U.S. empire (Escobar 2004; Quijano 2000, 227). It has also simultaneously involved looking to how nation-states maintained systems of social hierarchy and access to labor and resources, most centrally through projects of *mestizaje* (racial and cultural mixing) that sought to assimilate Indigenous and Black populations into whiteness[9]—a form of colonialism through the Latin American nation-state that some also discuss in terms of settler colonialism (Castellanos 2017; 2021; Speed 2017).[10]

In tracing the coloniality of Bolivian health care, I foreground how historical and contemporary dynamics of plunder have unequally distributed illness across sectors of society. Simultaneously, I emphasize how institutions created to address illness are rooted in a biopolitical project of regulating Indigenous life. This project has been essential, especially from the mid-twentieth century onwards, to Bolivian mestizo nation-state building and control over territory, even as it has also been sustained through transnational health programs and resource flows (see Pacino 2013; 2015).[11] Across multiple administrations, health policies have forwarded the racialization of Indigenous patient bodies as sources of pathology while positioning the adoption of biomedicine as a path to both modernization and social whitening. Echoing colonial biopolitical projects elsewhere (Million 2020; Morgensen 2011; Stevenson 2014), Bolivian health care provisions have also centrally revolved around remaking Indigenous and campesino lifeways in the name of sustaining biological, or bare, life. Health policies often positioned nonbiomedical ontologies of health and the body—for example, those rooted in relations with kin or with the surrounding landscape—as key targets of intervention and reform. Simultaneously, however, people's ability to "cooperate" in ostensibly life-saving projects (Stevenson 2014) was also undercut by the precariousness of institutional care in Bolivia: patchy state and transnational health infrastructures often meant that services were underresourced or difficult to access.

These histories have underpinned how health care contexts in Bolivia continue to be key sites of racialization and racial formation. More broadly, because of shifts in legal and political categories and layered histories of assimilation,[12] how people identify themselves and others is often context dependent. In Machacamarca, for example, while the vast majority of residents of the municipality of Machacamarca identified as Aymara on the census (Instituto Nacional de Estadística 2001; 2012), their use of terms such as *Indígena* (Indigenous) or, more rarely, *Indio* (Indian), also varied. Especially since the 1990s, as the term "Indígena" began to circulate more nationally and globally in association with emancipatory struggles, some town residents embraced it as a political identifier. Others, however, used it to refer to relatives who lived in more rural areas "as we did before." Still others preferred to use more class-based terms, distinguishing between rural *campesinos* (peasants) and urban *vecinos* (neighbors) who lived in the town center. Yet biomedical clinics also created specific sites for both enacting and entrenching racial formations. Emphasizing the malleability of conceptions of race in much of the Andean region, Elizabeth Roberts (2012) highlights how medical technologies—along with other material markers such as language, dress, and geographic origin—can racialize patients as more mestizo or more Indigenous. In the public hospital in Machacamarca, biomedical providers (including some whose parents or grandparents were Aymara rural-to-urban migrants) were often positioned as mestizo—or simply, unmarked—because of their professional and class status and access to biomedical knowledge. In turn, in biomedical encounters, both urban and rural residents of the municipality of Machacamarca were often racialized as Indigenous—that is, as patients who could rarely access the personalized attention of private care, who had to deal with long wait times and clinical resource shortages, and whom practitioners often presumed to be ignorant.

Still, as Indigenous Studies scholars have emphasized, indigeneity cannot be reduced only to an experience of colonization—not least because colonialism has never been a complete or totalizing process. To this end, many have called for centering the relations, knowledges, and practices that constitute indigeneity, in ways that also unsettle dominant legal, political, and scientific constructions (Arvin 2019;

Lambert 2022; TallBear 2013). In Machacamarca, long-standing relations with both human and other-than-human beings that formed the basis of healing have also never been fully subsumed into dominant approaches to health and medicine. Attending to the endurance of such relations does not mean treating them as pristine or unchanging over time, but it does highlight how relations—including localized projects of care and life-making—were continually refashioned and reasserted in new ways. These relations formed part of everyday practice, but also were at the center of wider conversations and debates in Bolivia about what a decolonial health policy might entail.

WARM CARE AT WORK

I first came to work in Machacamarca because state officials and NGO workers based in La Paz described the municipal hospital to me as an exemplar of decolonization and interculturality in health care. In the first six months of my long-term ethnographic fieldwork (from June to December 2014), I traced processes of health policymaking in the administrative capital of La Paz by interviewing state and regional health officials and attending planning meetings. During this period, I focused primarily on the bureaucratic practices and the production of state narratives about decolonization and health care reform. I also followed an NGO I give the pseudonym of "Global Health Aid," or GHA, on various day trips to sites across the Altiplano as they conducted workshops about national health policies. As I weighed various sites where I might more closely look at policy implementation for the next phase of my research (from January to December 2015), multiple officials suggested Machacamarca as a place where national health reforms were relatively well developed.

One of the reasons Machacamarca had become an exemplar was because long-standing state, municipal, and NGO collaborations in the municipality had already built up local health infrastructure. The hospital, constructed in 2001 with partial support from a European country's bilateral aid funding, served residents of the town and surrounding villages in the predominantly Aymara municipality. The location of the town of about eleven thousand residents was also attractive to aid organizations: a two-hour drive from La Paz, it was urbanized enough to have amenities like electricity, running water, and internet, yet still closely connected to numerous rural villages deemed in need of care and intervention (Figure I.1 and Figure I.2). Even before Evo Morales was elected president, municipal health services had worked with NGOs to foster collaborations between biomedical practitioners and Aymara traditional midwives and healers. These projects were then significantly expanded and reworked with the enactment of national health care reforms in the Morales era.

The trajectories that brought me—a white Swiss-Bolivian researcher affiliated with a university in the Global North—to Machacamarca closely followed the paths that brought numerous others to the highland Andean municipality. I joined a small trickle of other journalists and researchers writing about Bolivian health care reforms who had likewise passed through the town on similar recommendations. In positioning Machacamarca as an exemplar, state and NGO workers hoped to showcase the goals toward which they were working. Simultaneously, however, they frequently reflected on the challenges of putting policy into practice, describing implementation in Machacamarca and elsewhere as an unfinished work-in-progress.

As I came to understand, Bolivian state-led decolonization of health

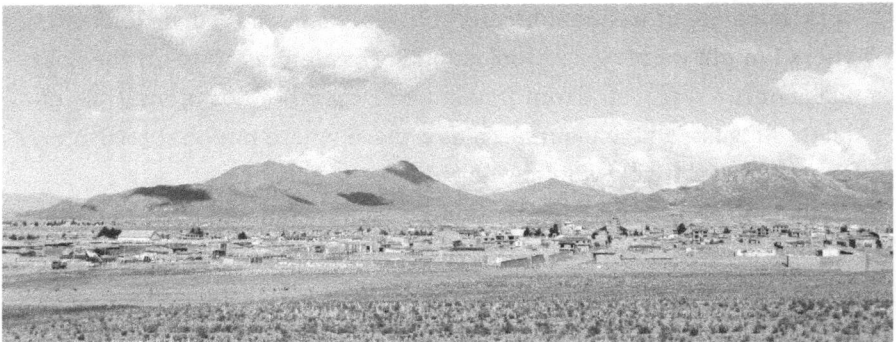

FIGURE I.1. Machacamarca from a distance. Source: Photograph by the author.

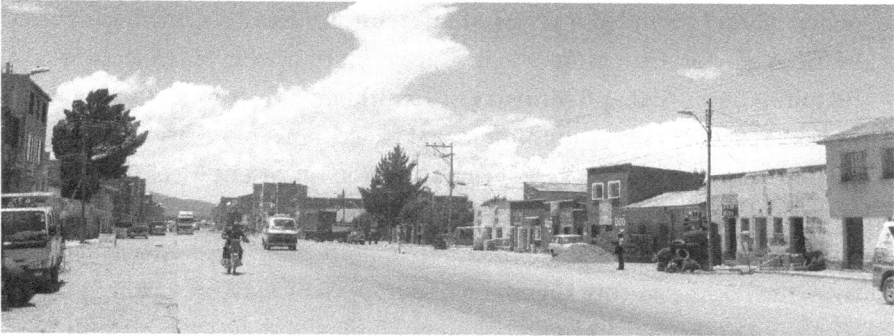

FIGURE I.2. The main highway that cuts through the town of Machacamarca. Source: Photograph by the author.

care was a contingent process, involving building up and rerouting existing infrastructures to implement new policies. For example, despite officials' stated hopes to decrease reliance on foreign aid organizations, they often worked closely with national and transnational NGOs to enact national health policies. Still, in contrast to the disaggregated forms of governmentality that often characterize aid projects under neoliberalism (Gupta and Sharma 2006; Nguyen 2010), NGOs operating in Bolivia during the Morales era often repositioned themselves as working continuously with the state. Emphasizing their technical experience and expertise, many organizations increasingly situated themselves as working to support the implementation of national policies and infrastructures (Cordoba and Jansen 2016). GHA, the main health NGO working in Machacamarca at the time of my research, was a well-known global organization with branches in many countries. While the Bolivian branch received its mandate from its parent organization in Europe, it was staffed entirely by Bolivians with backgrounds in sociology, education, and medicine. The nonprofit worked closely with Bolivian state officials to help implement reforms, including by running workshops and building new constructions such as culturally adapted birthing rooms and greenhouses at various clinics across the Altiplano, the Andean high plateau.

I was reminded of the labor and coordination needed to implement policy when I attended a series of intercultural health workshops run by GHA in 2015 for biomedical practitioners at the Machacamarca Hospital. Both NGO and Ministry of Health officials frequently offered workshops and courses for biomedical practitioners, traditional medical practitioners, and grassroots organization representatives. The goal of these didactic events was both to convey changes to national health policy and to encourage participants to shift their approach to care. Over the course of this specific workshop, GHA staffers running the meeting taught hospital practitioners about the definition of culture and provided several key examples of Aymara health beliefs and practices. They also explained the three main health care models described in an essay by anthropologist Eduardo Menéndez (1992): the hegemonic system; the alternative system; and home remedies. Interculturality, the NGO staffers explained, was an important tenet of the new national health policy: health establishments and providers should be working toward the "articulation and complementarity" between biomedical and traditional medical systems, the "cultural adaptation" of health services, and the strengthening of traditional medicine.

As the NGO staff members wrapped up their presentation, Alicia, the director of field operations for GHA, asked the workshop participants to share their own experiences engaging with patients' cultural beliefs. Many of the hospital providers commuted to work in Machacamarca from the cities of La Paz and El Alto; thus many of them were also unfamiliar with the local context until they began working at the hospital. A young practitioner named Dr. Estela volunteered that once she had treated a patient who came in with a gastrointestinal problem but was convinced that he had been attacked by a *kharikhari* (a monster that stole the fat from one's body). She was taken aback when the patient asked her to diagnose him as having been attacked by a kharikhari. Other providers jumped in to describe occasions when patients had not wanted to receive an injection because they had been victims of kharikharis. Several of those describing their experiences emphasized that interculturality in health care was all well and good, but there should be limits.

At this point, Alicia joined the conversation to assure the providers that she agreed with them. Interculturality was important, she stressed, but practices that were damaging for health should not be incorporated into the hospital setting.

The discussion was one of many I would encounter over the course of my research, as biomedical providers, NGO staffers, and state and regional health officials negotiated, debated, and tinkered with how to best care for an Indigenous patient population. "Culture"—usually understood as a bounded, static marker of Indigenous difference—was often the basis for conversations about providing for others. Echoing wider dynamics of liberal recognition politics (Povinelli 2002), institutional actors' negotiations often entailed drawing boundaries around what kinds of practices were commensurate with hospital practice and which ones were deemed too threatening to life itself—although providers, NGO staffers, and state and regional officials sometimes had differing ideas about where the line should be drawn. Simultaneously, these negotiations around cultural inclusion were tied to new forms of attention: through formats like the workshop, providers were encouraged to provide care *con calidad y calidez*, to treat patients humanely and equally, and to be sensitive to difference even while working within a biomedical frame. These were the kinds of practices that came to characterize what I think of as warm care.

In national policy documents, discussions of decolonization and interculturality in health care often went beyond a focus on warmth and cultural sensitivity. Drawing from Indigenous and decolonial activist projects, Bolivian state reformers proposed a system that would move beyond treatment of the biological body and instead foreground Indigenous conceptions of health grounded in relations with "family, community, and nature" (Ministerio de Salud y Deportes 2008, 20, my translation). They also proposed the construction of a radically pluralist health system, in which Indigenous traditional medical practitioners might work alongside biomedical doctors and in which patients might choose multiple options of care (Bernstein 2017; Johnson 2010).

Yet if activist proposals for decolonization often centered a process of unsettling and undoing, in practice, state, medical, and nonprofit institutions struggled to hold tension. One easy read of the interculturality workshop might be that the transnational NGO was reinterpreting state policies in ways that aligned with models of interculturality within regional and global health—thereby watering down the more radically disruptive proposals written into Bolivian state policy texts. However, while it was the case that the NGO brought its own approach to state policies, it was not the only institution to do so; state, regional, and local health officials, as well as hospital providers, all tinkered with policies in different but overlapping ways, often with the goal of rendering plural health practices and ontologies commensurate with existing biomedical forms. Building on my conversations with bureaucrats, providers, and patients, I trace how elements of health policy designed to subvert the status quo (for example, via a focus on relational conceptions of health and the emphasis on parity of knowledge systems) were folded into a practice of warm care that maintained existing colonial structures.

Understanding this subsuming process as tied to care, I suggest, is particularly helpful.[13] For Medical Anthropology and Science and Technology Studies (STS) scholars writing about care, care might be best understood capaciously—as a form of "providing for others" (Aulino 2019, 5) or "the way someone comes to matter and the corresponding ethics of attending to the other who matters" (Stevenson 2014, 3). As an analytic, care draws attention to the variety of ways individuals, communities, and institutions engage questions of who should be provided for and how.[14] Importantly, care can also move between dominant and resistive forms; it can work to sustain social hierarchies and to undo them (Matza 2018). Analyzing care as an integral component of colonial projects means attending to how institutions have invoked benevolence when providing for colonized subjects, while furthering control over Indigenous land, labor, knowledges, and lifeways. It also highlights how institutional projects might seek to assimilate, monitor, or intervene in nonhegemonic relations of care, even as they never fully succeed in erasing them (Million 2020).

Examining how global reproductive rights organizations mobilize care, particularly in interventions geared toward the Global South, Métis STS scholar Michelle Murphy cautions against conflating "care with affection, happiness, attachment, and positive feeling as political goods" (2015, 719). Calling for a focus on care's "non-innocent genealogies," Murphy traces how good feelings can operate in support of hegemonic structures: "This vexation of care is important because there is an ongoing temptation within feminist scholarship to view positive affect and care as a route to emancipated science and alternative knowledge-making without critically examining the ways positive feelings, sympathy, and other forms of attachment can work with and through the grain of hegemonic structures, rather than against them" (719). Thus projects of care and compassion—at least when mobilized through dominant institutions—can also operate as an "antipolitics" that forecloses structural change (Ticktin 2011). While writing less directly about care, others have likewise noted how liberal settler states' projects of reconciliation mobilize good feelings of sympathy (Simpson 2020) and promise to build a "kinder, gentler society" (Million 2013, 50); these affective moves ultimately depoliticize and deny Indigenous claims to self-determination.

Such works offer an important basis for understanding how, in the Bolivian context, warm care—as an affective, ontological, material, and ethical mode of providing for others—extended colonial dynamics. Warm care, I suggest, kept intact colonial biopolitical projects to monitor, regulate, and intervene in Indigenous bodies and populations. In fact, under Morales-era health reforms, disciplinary technologies expanded in scope, as health officials developed new bureaucratic mechanisms for collecting data on rural household practices, mapping community risk factors, regulating Indigenous healing and midwifery practices, and more. These bureaucratic mechanisms positioned rural, Indigenous, and low-income populations as racialized sources of risk, whose cultural practices needed to be regulated and managed in the name of sustaining life itself. Yet warm care tied these biopolitical interventions to new forms of inclusion, kindness, and gentle attention. It became a modality through which bureaucrats and medical providers attended to the perceived cultural difference of Indigenous patients, while also rendering that difference commensurate with biomedical and biopolitical modes of intervention.

Even as warmth extended state care in new directions, it also fore-closed other possibilities of care. Take, for example, the kharikhari, which the biomedical providers in the workshop described as an-tithetical to biomedical diagnosis and a source of patient refusal. Kharikharis (also called *karisiris* or *pishtacos* elsewhere in the Andes) manifested bodily extraction: often appearing in the guise of a white outsider, the kharikhari stole the fat (one's life force) from unsuspect-ing individuals. Anthropologists working with Andean Indigenous communities have often pointed to the kharikhari as a local theori-zation of colonial and capitalist extraction, as well as a violation of moral norms centered on reciprocity and mutual obligation (Aber-crombie 1998; Canessa 2012; Weismantel 2001). Among residents of Machacamarca, however, the very existence of the kharikhari was also contested. Rural urbanization and shifting ontologies of health and illness prompted some of my interlocutors to wonder out loud if the kharikhari even existed. Others suggested that perhaps it was not fat that the kharikhari stole, but blood, for they had seen bags of blood in the hospital.[15] Residents of Machacamarca, in short, often disagreed on the nature of the kharikhari, or whether it existed at all. For some, the kharikhari remained a powerful (and yet ontologically unstable) being emerging from extractive medical practices in the hospital. Yet as institutional actors weighed the kharikhari primarily as a uniform cultural belief that should or should not be incorporated under new paradigms of inclusion, they foreclosed other relational possibilities opened up by the kharikhari. If some town residents wor-ried the kharikhari emerged in a context of extraction, they also hoped that providers might engage in care more centered on relationships of mutual obligation. For many, establishing relations of exchange with providers—in which providers were expected to attend to patients in the long term, to be imbricated in patients' social and moral worlds—could restore bodily health and well-being. In this book, I dwell on how warm care not only flattened more radical proposals for decoloniza-tion, but also partially foreclosed more accountable engagements with patients' contexts and worlds.

STATE-LED DECOLONIZATION

When Evo Morales, the Aymara leader of a major coca growers' union, was first elected president of Bolivia in 2005, he vowed to undertake a project of decolonizing the nation-state, invoking the intertwined apparatuses of colonialism and capitalism that continued to maintain the oppression of the Indigenous and poor. State discourses of decolonization often emerged in highly visible public sites–for example, through rituals like the inauguration of President Morales at the archaeological ruins of Tiwanaku, or through the installation of a backwards clock on the presidential palace to disrupt Eurocentric paradigms of linear time. But it was also a framework that appeared across multiple policy and bureaucratic texts, shaping policy across a range of fields, including health care, education, land reform, the judicial system, and foreign policy. Shortly after Morales took office, his administration put forward its National Development Plan, designed to guide state approaches to policy across the board. In a section titled "The Route to Decolonize the State from the State," the plan stated directly,

> The proposal for the new institutionality of the Bolivian State consists in taking on its own decolonization from within its own structures, practices, and discourses. The colonial composition of the state apparatus and the urgency of dismantling the explicit and implicit mechanisms that connote and denote this coloniality is due to the ways [this coloniality] is impregnated in the structure of the State and its daily functions. The continual reconstruction of the colonial penetrated all social spheres and within this were mixed elements of domination, ethnic exclusion, racism, and hegemony, mystified by the liberal and neoliberal modernization of segments of society. (Ministerio de Planificación del Desarollo 2007: 14, my translation)

Drawing from the work long undertaken by Indigenous movements and public intellectuals in Bolivia, the National Development Plan drew attention to the continual reinscription of colonialism and its embeddedness in the very structures of the state. But what did it look like in practice for the state to undertake "its own decolonization from within its own structures, practices, and discourses"? How did this project come to shape approaches to medical care and health policy?

When I started working on this project in 2012 and began sharing research proposals with others, I received a number of responses from colleagues and reviewers based in the United States who expressed confusion about what "decolonization" entailed—or surprise that Bolivian officials would use a term primarily associated with a period of post–World War II nation-state formation. However, in the years since then, the term "decolonization" has become seemingly ubiquitous in academic circles. Its use has become increasingly widespread in institutional spaces and fields of knowledge production, particularly as it has become mainstreamed in the Global North. Calls for decolonization, for example, have emerged within fields of medicine, science, and global health to reckon with historically entrenched inequalities and exclusions.[16] Humanistic and social science research has been described as currently going through a "decolonial turn." That is, if Indigenous, Black, and subaltern movements have long undertaken a range of projects—across a range of contexts and timescales—to dismantle colonial apparatuses, there has been an increasing turn (seemingly) to thinking *within* dominant spaces about how to reckon with oppressive legacies and presents.

At the same time, the growing institutional use of this framing has also raised concerns that decolonization has become metaphorical or equivalent to "diversity, equity, and inclusion," rather than entailing the material reversal of colonial processes of domination and dispossession (Tuck and Yang 2012; Todd 2015). As Eve Tuck and Wayne Yang have powerfully argued, decolonization "is not a generic term for struggle against oppressive conditions and outcomes. . . . [It] specifically requires the repatriation of Indigenous land and life" (2012, 21). Concerns about the limits of institution-led decolonization have also emerged in the interrelated fields of science, medicine, and public and global health. Attentive to decolonization's demands for structural undoing, Seye Abimbola and Madhukar Pai directly ask, "Will global health survive its decolonization?" (2020, 1627). It might, they suggest—but only if its practitioners "commit to its transformation" (1627) through antisupremacist and antiracist practice. In the environmental and lab sciences, Max Liboiron echoes Tuck and Yang's insistence that decolonization entails nothing short of the return of Indigenous land and life—and prefers to take up the term "anticolonial" to describe methods that "do not reproduce settler and colonial entitlement to Land and Indigenous cultures, concepts, knowledges (including Traditional Knowledge), and lifeworlds" (2021, 27). These vital conversations and critiques point to the multiplicity of work toward transformation—as well as the ways projects of liberal inclusion might deflect from or co-opt this work.

In Bolivia, where state moves to decolonization slightly predated the term's global mainstreaming, activists and intellectuals have expressed resonant preoccupations about superficial institutional appropriations of the term "decolonization" (Portugal Mollinedo 2011; Rivera Cusicanqui 2014). Nonetheless, I also want to be careful to avoid conflating conversations about decolonization in Bolivia with conversations happening elsewhere around the globe. Bolivian institutional efforts emerged from situated activist genealogies and took shape amid a national politics that, if not exactly socialist, was moving toward state-led redistribution and public investment. Attending to institutional processes in Bolivia illuminates how proposals for transformation move from activist circles to bureaucratic policymaking to implementation in multiple, nonlinear, and entangled ways. In this text, I think with ongoing debates in Bolivia about the possibilities and limits of this institutional transformation.

Actions toward and debates about decolonization in Bolivia are wide-ranging and multivocal; I do not cover all of them here. But I point, especially, to ongoing debates among Aymara and Quechua activists and scholars[17] as well as allied communities about whether the state could be a vehicle for decolonization. As members of the intellectual collective Grupo Comuna argued, the state was a "battlefield" (*campo de lucha*), where questions of its reproduction and transformation were always in question (García Linera, Tapia, Vega, and Prada 2010).

Broadly, one historical line of decolonial thought emphasized the abolition of the Bolivian state as a fundamentally colonial institution, governed by a European-descended minority, that maintained conditions of Indigenous oppression across multiple sites. Perhaps most influentially, the Aymara activist and political theorist Fausto Reinaga called for a "struggle of national liberation" (1969, 442, my translation) to overturn the white-mestizo-ruled state and colonial order. Thinking both with and against Marxist currents, he grew disenchanted with the limits of Marxist conceptions of revolution for Indian struggle. He called for a shedding of Eurocentric conceptions and a centering of Indian cosmologies to build a more just society. In the 1970s, members of the Aymara-led Indianista-Katarista intellectual and political movement directly drew on Reinaga's writings to call for the abolition of the colonial state and reconstitution of the Tawatinsuyu (the Incan realm) (Choque Canqui 2010; Dangl 2019; Sanjinés 2004). But this project of articulating political worlds outside the state also emerged across multiple other sites, in other forms. The work undertaken by the Andean Oral History Workshop (*Taller de Historia Oral Andina,* THOA) demonstrated how communitarian and anarchist thought had long been central to Indigenous and popular struggle in Bolivia (Lehm Ardaya and Rivera Cusicanqui 1988). Building in part from work undertaken by the THOA, the National Council of Ayllus and Markas of Qullasuyu, an Aymara, Quechua, and Uru movement, formed in the 1990s to restore the *ayllu,* a kin-based system of communal governance that had once been central to the organization of Andean Indigenous communities. Many members of the movement pointed to the persistence of forms of rotational labor, reciprocal practice, and other forms of the communal as having resisted colonial attempts at eradication—and positioned the restoration of the ayllu as part of a project to ultimately restore Indigenous good living.

Others, in turn, proposed not so much the rejection of the state form as a profound restructuring of relations between citizen, state, and society. Yet these positions were not completely separate from more anarchist or abolitionist lines of thought; rather, there was considerable debate and cross-fertilization across these perspectives. Aymara activists and members of the THOA Maria Eugenia Choque and Carlos Mamani (2001) argued, for example, for a deepening of a pluralist state, in which Indigenous communities would both have the power of self-determination for their own nation and be able to engage in dialogue on equal footing (rather than in a subordinate position) with those who were descended from the colonial invaders. Others, like Félix Patzi Paco (2004), an Aymara sociologist who became minister of education under Morales, argued that the ayllu itself was the basis of a communal politics that should inform the remaking of the colonial state—a state that itself would be decolonized through an emphasis on pluriversalism, reciprocity, and abundant redistribution. Carrying echoes of Reinaga's earlier work, activists articulated notions of the communal that were in part resonant with and in alliance with other leftist projects (that were calling for redistribution and critiquing capitalist exploitation), but also situated this as coming from a specifically Indigenous world-making project (Mignolo 2010).

Although the Morales administration clearly took the stance that, yes, the state could self-decolonize, it drew from multiple genealogies to articulate its project of decolonization. As Mark Goodale (2019, 217) describes, Morales administration officials also handed out copies of Fausto Reinaga's *La Revolución India* (*The Indian Revolution*) (1969) at events and positioned themselves as the inheritors of his project to recenter Indigenous ontologies as the basis for a more just society. Broadly, moves toward state-led decolonization revolved around two key goals. First was the notion that state policies might be guided by an Indigenous relational ethics to guarantee "good living"—usually glossed in Spanish as *Vivir Bien* and sometimes also referred to as *Suma Qamaña* in Aymara and *Sumak Kawsay* in Quechua. Policymakers and advocates positioned Vivir Bien as stemming from principles of collective well-being and harmonious relations with both human and other-than-human communities; these ethical orientations, moreover, would offer a substantive alternative to a colonial and capitalist extractive system of *vivir mejor* (living better) (Albó 2009; Choquehuanca 2010; Huanacuni 2010). Second was a focus on supporting epistemological and ontological pluralism—in which, for example, Indigenous knowledge-practices might be incorporated into the health care, judicial, and educational systems (Johnson 2010; Patzi Paco 2014). This approach was echoed in the rewriting of the Bolivian constitution, which established Bolivia as a plurinational state—that is, a state made up of thirty-six officially recognized nations that could also exercise cultural and territorial autonomy, albeit still within the ambit of the centralized state (Postero 2017; Regalsky 2009; Schavelzón 2012).

The paradigm of decolonization came to shape a large range of Morales-era policies. Turning specifically to projects to decolonize the health care system, I center on the making and implementation of two key policies. The Family, Community, and Intercultural Health (*Salud Familiar Comunitaria e Intercultural*, SAFCI) policy, enacted in 2008, centered the creation of a health care system that combined tenets of social medicine (such as equality of access and an emphasis on primary and preventative community-based care) with those of interculturality (including recognizing plural knowledge systems) (Bernstein 2017; Johnson 2010). State officials described the law as a "new way of feeling, thinking, understanding, and doing health" that would also be based in an Indigenous relational ethics of Vivir Bien. In doing so, it would offer an alternative to strictly treatment-based models of biomedicine to instead foreground "relations with family, community, and nature" as a central component of health (Ministerio de Salud y Deportes 2008, 20, my translation). Building from this earlier Morales administration policy, the Law of Traditional and Ancestral Medicine (*Ley de Medicina Tradicional Ancestral*), passed in 2013, instated a system for regulating and credentialing the practice of traditional medicine, significantly expanding the protections of prior legalization efforts (Babis 2014; 2018). As with the SAFCI, Bolivian state officials situated the law as part of a move toward decolonizing health care that would place multiple knowledge systems on equal footing within institutions.

Significantly, Morales administration officials distinguished health and other decolonizing reforms from policies of neoliberal multicultural recognition that had come before. In the 1990s, in response to national and global Indigenous rights movements, President Gonzalo Sánchez de Lozada enacted policies to extend new rights and cultural recognition to Indigenous peoples, albeit on limited terms. Policies included measures such as popular participation, bilingual education, and, in the realm of health care, some initial efforts to integrate Indigenous traditional medicine and home birthing into clinical settings. These policies unfolded alongside neoliberal economic reforms that also deepened many inequalities and put Indigenous and impoverished Bolivians in a precarious position (Albro 2010; Gustafson 2009b). Nancy Postero (2007) argues that frustration with the limitations of neoliberal multiculturalism prompted Morales's political party, the MAS, to both promise a deepening of Indigenous rights and embrace a more redistributive economic model. For many officials I interviewed, the framework of decolonization went further than prior models of rights and recognition, laying the groundwork for remaking existing state structures to be oriented toward Indigenous good living. For them, "the route to decolonize the State from the State" entailed thinking with Indigenous cosmologies as the basis for reshaping institutions from within and imagining a more just and equitable society.

POLITICAL ECONOMIES OF REINSCRIPTION

Over the course of Morales's nearly fourteen years in office, however, the scope of decolonial reforms grew more limited, prompting commentary, critique, and complaint among many I interviewed. According to at least some policymakers who had previously worked on the SAFCI policy, the Morales administration, especially in the president's later terms, had given the policy lower priority in favor of others, like new hospital constructions. For many patients and healers living in Machacamarca, day-to-day experiences in the hospital continued to be a site of "no care"—where policies to promote inclusion (such as culturally adapted birthing rooms) were sometimes seen as beneficial, but as not going far enough. As I work to understand the limitations and reinscriptions that took shape through state-led decolonization of the health care system, my goal is not to deny the importance of projects to challenge colonial and neoliberal capitalist configurations, both within and beyond the state form. Rather, my goal is to understand why and how a far-reaching vision of transformation articulated by activists, bureaucrats, and very often in policy texts was folded into a practice of warm care that maintained the status quo.

Reinscriptions that unfolded in health policy were continuous with other, wider tensions that took shape within the Bolivian state's decolonial project. Most visible, perhaps, were tensions that emerged as Bolivian state projects of extractive development—in which investment and taxation on oil and gas industries might fund public infrastructure projects—eroded its promised strengthening of Indigenous sovereignty (Anthias 2018; Calla 2020; Gustafson 2020; Postero 2017). Other tensions also began to emerge. While the MAS continued to enjoy support among many Indigenous, labor, and populist movements, some argued that the party had ultimately backtracked on its commitments to them—for example, as it adopted watered-down versions of movement proposals for the constitution or made concessions to lowland agribusiness (Postero 2017; Goodale 2019). Thus whether the state had succeeded in acting as a vehicle for change or whether it had simply co-opted movement language while maintaining the status quo continued to be a point of ongoing discussion among Indigenous and worker movements in Bolivia (Calla 2020; Rivera Cusicanqui 2014). Aymara public intellectuals such as Carlos Macusaya Cruz (2014) and Pedro Portugal Mollinedo (2011) argued that the Morales administration was deepening a politics that romanticized Indigenous difference while offering Indigenous peoples little real justice or transformation. Others, in turn, emphasized that the MAS did achieve many concrete goals that transformed lives for the better: rising standards of living, new antidiscrimination and gender parity laws, popular conditional cash transfer programs, and much needed public infrastructures continued to make Evo Morales a popular president.

Scholars working in Bolivia have suggested that some of the contradictions, fragmentations, and dilutions that took shape within the MAS's decolonial project need to be understood in connection to the limitations of the liberal settler state as a vehicle for change. As the MAS shifted from a project of "emancipation to one of liberal nation-state building" (Postero 2017, 5), it largely maintained an existing capitalist economy and state legislative system, even as it sought to reroute these to achieve goals the Morales administration put forward (Postero 2017; Goodale 2019; Grisaffi 2019; Winchell 2022). More broadly, scholars have argued that liberalism—reflecting Enlightenment ideals of rationality, progress, and individual freedom—cannot be separated from the historical rise of "colonialism, slavery, capitalism, and empire" (Lowe 2015, 4) that positioned European Man as the locus of rationality, civilization, and the human (Wynter 2003). Policy efforts to extend legal rights and protections in new directions—for example, under liberal multiculturalism and recognition politics—continue to maintain, rather than challenge, dominant structures of carcerality and dispossession (Coulthard 2014; Povinelli 2002; Shange 2019; Simpson 2014). In the Bolivian context, scholars have likewise highlighted how channeling decolonial proposals through liberal mechanisms of government constrained possibilities of change. Mareike Winchell (2020; 2022) argues, for example, that MAS policies intended to emancipate Quechua farmers relied on the liberal presuppositions of earlier land reforms, positioning both colonial systems and Indigenous kinship practices as equally irrational. Penelope Anthias locates the "limits to decolonization" in the MAS's ongoing reliance—despite statements otherwise—on paradigms of cultural recognition, first implemented under the neoliberal state of the 1990s. She argues that projects of recognition were not confined to a single administration, but "always conditioned by colonial knowledge-power inequalities and settler interests in indigenous territory and resources" (2018, 10).

Like other scholars working on the Morales era in Bolivia, I have found it relevant to turn to the limitations of enacting change through the liberal state form. Warm care, I suggest, emerged in part out of a liberal paradigm of inclusion. Providing for others was tied to acknowledging Indigenous patients' cultural difference through partial engagements with their worlds and through gentle and warm affects. But it was primarily oriented around making difference manageable and bringing it into the fold of dominant state and biomedical systems. However, where I differ slightly from others who have written about liberalism and the MAS is in my focus on the relationship between liberalism and unequal flows of resources and labor that conditioned the provision of public services. Warm care, I suggest, required resources and labor to maintain, but also became a means to deflect from how these dynamics continued to constrain the health care system.

Resources presented a central paradox of state care under Evo Morales. While the MAS largely maintained a capitalist system, it vowed to reinvest wealth from natural resource extraction into social infrastructures, cash bonuses, and other projects of state care that would distinguish it from predecessors' neoliberal austerity. Yet if the Morales administration did increase health care spending,[18] the new regimes of state extractivism were not sufficient to overturn decades of state underfunding, neocolonial global resource flows, and patchy infrastructures for health care delivery. The landscape of Bolivian health care in practice remained fragmentary, as the Ministry of Health continued to rely on nonprofit organizations to help with implementing public policies, and as private and employer insurance schemes remained preferred options for patients who could afford them. In pointing out ongoing conditions of fragmentation and underfunding, I do not suggest that state officials should have extracted even more resources from lowland Indigenous territories to fuel national services. Rather, conditions were already rigged to reproduce inequalities: the promise of popular health care was still predicated on colonial extraction, still operated within a global capitalist system, still shaped by national and global conditions that came before.

Amid resource constraints in the health care system, the sustenance of warm care relied heavily on un- and undercompensated labor of those deemed closer to "patient culture," such as Aymara midwives and traditional healers. While norms varied by municipality, many healers and midwives (including those based in the Machacamarca Hospital) did not receive salaries when working in clinical settings. Within regimes of limited institutional funding, Indigenous midwives and healers were often given low priority. Most officials I interviewed agreed on principle that traditional practitioners should be systematically paid, but they had not instated formal mechanisms for ensuring that they would be. Yet midwife and healer labor was also central to sustaining institutional projects of warm care: they were often expected to do the work of cultural translation, to show kindness to patients, and to bring more patients into the clinic. For healers and midwives themselves, participation in this system (even without pay) remained an important path to prestige and to legitimating their practice, particularly in a context in which the state had historically criminalized their work. They refigured institutional projects to reflect their own approaches, exceeding the paradigm of warm care by restoring patient relations with human and other-than-human beings. And yet, in practice, their labor was also appropriated to sustain much of the daily functioning of warm care in the hospital.

Attending to questions of resources, funding, and labor is important because it highlights the broader structural dynamics that continue to shape not only the incidence of illness but also the conditions of care itself. Contestations over how resources should be used in medical contexts were inseparable from global dynamics of privatization and aid, as well as from the Bolivian state's turn to resources to reassert national sovereignty. These, too, were extensions of deep-rooted colonial and capitalist dynamics, at both the global and national levels. But if Bolivian state bureaucrats—and policy texts themselves—frequently referenced problems of colonialism and capitalism, they positioned their solutions in limited terms of liberal inclusion, affective warmth, and kindness. As reformers continued to enact change within existing state and medical apparatuses, warm care became a way to maintain existing infrastructures, coordinations, and ways of approaching health that had long made health care hang together, however imperfectly, as a biopolitical system. Simultaneously, warm care—as both an institutional discourse and an everyday practice in medical contexts—worked to obfuscate and deflect from enduring structural inequalities. For example, it could simultaneously entrench racializing dynamics of patient care, while (through the invocation of good feelings) also obfuscating the very existence of racial hierarchies and material inequalities in the clinic. Warm care also underpinned the recruitment of Indigenous healers and midwives, as institutions extended promises of inclusion; yet these very promises of inclusion were also leveraged to offset healers' concerns around compensation.

TROUBLING MATTERS OF CARE

Although I first came to live in Machacamarca through my connections with state and NGO workers, I came to spend considerable time outside of formal institutional settings. I lodged with a family in town and got to know residents of both the town and surrounding villages. When I was not working in the hospital, I regularly helped with chores like planting, harvesting, sheepherding, and selling goods at the local market. Residents of the municipality expected me to follow through on my ethical obligations to them, particularly given my position as someone with greater resources at my disposal. Obligations included presenting on my research, as well as sharing in food and labor, returning for visits, and, on some occasions, becoming a godmother to children. Forging ties of kinship did not erase social hierarchies but became a key means to hold me (and others) accountable to long-term obligations across these hierarchies (Leinaweaver 2008; Winchell 2022).

Such forms of accountability also shaped many of my interlocutors' engagements with state and medical projects. Mareike Winchell (2022) notes that rural Andeans have long expected powerful actors to provide for others as a fulfillment of their moral obligations—a form of ethical accountability across hierarchies that, she argues, many also came to expect from the Morales administration. For Winchell, these notions of accountability underpin what many understand to be appropriate expressions of authority versus inappropriate ones. Building on this work, I show how my interlocutors emphasized state and medical institutions' obligations toward patients, particularly in a context in which many residents of Machacamarca felt that through their political activism, they had directly helped bring Evo Morales and the MAS to the presidency. While some of my interlocutors refused engagement with state and medical institutions entirely, for many others, relations of obligation were a means to hold the Bolivian state accountable to its promises and shape its trajectory of action (including, for some, in ways that still held to the aspirational project of the MAS). For example, uncompensated healers positioned state obligations to redistribute resources as essential to healing relationships that had been ruptured through urbanization, alienation, and labor precarity. Many patients, in turn, asked biomedical providers to become godparents, understanding kin relations to be an ontological ground for constituting health and well-being. Machacamarqueños often worked within existing social hierarchies to demand accountability, building on wider and long-standing forms of kin-making and patronage that figured into the moral norms of everyday life in the rural Andes (Winchell 2022).

Through conversation with my interlocutors, I came to understand such expectations as a continued partial engagement with state projects. Aymara residents of the municipality of Machacamarca sometimes desired aspects of warm care—for example, as patients requested use of the culturally adapted room, as healers and midwives asserted their right to practice in the hospital, and as patients lodged complaints about practitioners' mistreatment. Violeta's joking commentary that opened this introduction pointed to a desire for care that was promised but not fulfilled—highlighting how some patients might welcome multilingual care that functioned in practice. Simultaneously, my interlocutors refigured institutional projects of care through local ethical norms. As others have argued, people rarely internalize biopolitical subjectivities directly—but may creatively rework them (Brotherton 2012) or refract them through other relations (Han 2012). In Machacamarca, relations of ethical obligation among both human and other-than-human beings became a central ground for redefining institutional projects toward other ends of care. These forms of obligation and accountability subverted the ontological separations that still underpinned warm care—for example, between practitioners and patients, between bodies and landscapes—and instead positioned relations among various entities as central to constituting health and illness.

In other instances, when institutions' obligations to patients appeared to fall through entirely, residents of Machacamarca developed critiques of the state through practices of contention and complaint. Complaining (renegando) about state services (including health services) was sometimes an intimate practice between confidants, or a response to a moment of mistreatment in the hospital. But it could also take on public forms, as complaining became a common practice of speech-making in civil society spaces and forums for popular participation. As others have noted, practices like resentment, contention, and complaint are key resources and modes of engagement when countering the workings of liberal settler institutions (Ahmed 2021; Coulthard 2014; Simpson 2016). Likewise, I turn to practices of complaint to engage how residents of Machacamarca pushed beyond the limits of warm care, including its demands for commensuration and collaboration.

If warm care often foreclosed possibilities for transformation, practices of obligation and complaint raised questions about care as a site of political transformation and repair. Engaging with genealogies of Black and Indigenous feminist thought, scholars have suggested that relations of care can be central to what Aisha Finch describes as "a deliberate and purposeful creation of collective well-being" (2022, 2) that carves out spaces for radical alterity that reject colonial and capitalist orders.[19] As Hi'ilei Hobart and Tamara Kneese (2020) argue, if care can be co-opted or take on oppressive forms, it can also carry radical possibilities for survival and crafting worlds otherwise, particularly amid institutional failure and neglect. As they put it, "Reciprocity and attentiveness to the inequitable dynamics that characterize our current social landscape represent the kind of care that can radically remake our worlds that exceed those offered by the neoliberal or postneoliberal state, which has proved inadequate in its dispensation of care" (2020, 3). Care is not necessarily a replacement for other forms of political action, but it can be continuous with them, a terrain, even, for articulating them—a form, as Felicity Aulino suggests, of "plodding the revolution" (2019, 17).

The question then becomes not whether care is inherently resistive or oppressive, but rather how and when it is enacted—and under what terms. For many people I interviewed in Machacamarca, building more habitable worlds often entailed hard, burdensome care work—work that could also involve tactics of resentment and complaint, as well as the continuous, unfinished work of creating accountability across hierarchies. Attending to this work was important because state, biomedical, and nonprofit actors often mobilized the seemingly warm, positive, good feeling aspects of care to shut down complaint—to imply, "We care, you are being included, you should be grateful." Practices of obligation and complaint became a means to reroute care toward other goals of well-being. As I came to understand through conversations with town residents, these practices were oriented not only around what might make care better or constitute well-being in the moment, but also toward the wider conditions that might enable thriving more broadly. When enacted to fulfill ethical obligations, institutional care might entail more equitable resource distribution, move beyond inclusion to tackle racism, and forge modes of healing that did not demand commensuration with dominant norms. For many of my interlocutors, state and medical institutions continued to be sources of profound ambivalence. Through their engagements with care, they continually demanded more from the state than effusions of good feeling and nominal inclusion.

STRUCTURE OF THE BOOK

In keeping with its methodological and theoretical commitments, the structure of this book moves from the centers of policymaking in La Paz to implementation in Machacamarca.

Chapter 1 contextualizes the making of Bolivian health policy. In doing so, it centers questions of when Indigenous worlds were recognized, when they were erased entirely, and on what terms they were invoked to reshape care. Tracking bureaucratic practices across state and regional governing institutions, as well as nonprofit organizations, I highlight a multiplicity of projects and efforts that invoked the promise of descolonización. My interest lies in tracing how, amid this multiplicity, a paradigm of warm care came to dominate state proposals for transformation. I show how this iteration of care became a key site of commensuration between projects, including in ways that facilitated alignment with regional and global health models. Yet while warmth articulated aspirational horizons for Indigenous good living, it largely maintained forms of fixing, improvement, and hierarchy that had long been embedded in health care provision. While highlighting the nuance of policymakers' negotiations and efforts to rethink care, I illuminate the stickiness of coloniality through projects of state transformation.

Each of the five subsequent chapters takes up a different element of policy as it is enacted in Machacamarca: reorienting biomedical practice, cultural adaptation, the incorporation of traditional healing, community health work, and popular participation. Rather than simply describing policy implementation, this book takes each of these elements as a problem to think with.

Chapter 2 centers state efforts to "reorient" biomedical care via training courses and workshops that encouraged biomedical providers to incorporate moral practices of equality, kindness, and attentiveness into their work. For many biomedical practitioners in the Machacamarca Hospital, workshops became spaces where they could role-play an ideal form of care provision, in which all patients would be treated equally (and where the perpetual challenges of resource shortages were seemingly not a factor). Yet in everyday hospital practice, doctors and nurses often continued to treat patients paternalistically or harshly, leading many patients to describe their hospital experience as one of "no care." Puzzling through this tension between aspiration and practice, this chapter situates hospital care within a deeper lineage of state and medical violence, as well as within layered histories of material scarcity and constraint. I show how, as biomedical practitioners came to embrace "warm" ideals of kindness and equality, they did not displace older, harsh forms of care; rather, they enacted multiple moral and material projects in tandem.

Following closely on the heels of the second chapter, Chapter 3 examines another effort to decolonize the conditions of biomedical care in the Machacamarca Hospital: the construction of culturally adapted birthing rooms—warm, orange-hued rooms, equipped with beds and a small kitchen to invoke the homes where many Aymara women preferred to give birth. Warm aesthetics and built environment became central to promises of good care in the hospital. Attending to ontologies of temperature, I describe how, during home births, residents of Machacamarca often attended to the cold as a lively, potentially dangerous force that could cause sickness or death of the laboring mother. Yet in the hospital birthing rooms, institutional actors enacted warmth, not as a matter of life and death, but rather in terms of invitation, inclusivity, and "psychological support." While this mobilization of warm matter and practice at times enabled new forms of intimate care during hospital birth, it also extended racializing logics that positioned culture as a threat to be managed.

Chapter 4 shifts the focus to decolonial policy initiatives to certify traditional healers and invite them to work in hospitals and clinics. It foregrounds a central tension: even as they were granted new professional legitimacy, traditional practitioners who worked in clinical settings were rarely paid for their labor. This chapter examines how healers situated state institutions alongside human and other-than-human relations that could either sustain or impede patient well-being; they vocally demanded that the state materially invest in salaries, supplies, and maintenance to nourish relations essential to healing. Through anticipatory practices and forms of claims-making, healers redefined state promises of redistribution as a moral obligation to care for embodied relations and counter the illness-inducing effects of alienation.

Building on the theme of holding institutions accountable to promises, Chapter 5 turns to how patients worked to refigure biomedical care through lines of kinship and obligation. Under conditions of uncertain medical care, some residents of Machacamarca asked hospital practitioners to become godparents of their children. I read patient-initiated kinship practices critically against state efforts to move care out of the hospital and into the wider community. Efforts to create holistic and preventative care invoked the language of Indigenous relationality, but also subjected kin relations to biopolitical surveillance and monitoring of those deemed pathological threats to health. This chapter demonstrates how patient-initiated kin-work strove to refigure the colonial hospital in terms of intimacy and obligation, rather than monitoring and surveillance. It centers the forms of obligation, redistribution, and accountability across hierarchies that Machacamarqueños articulated through engagements with and against state promises of warm care.

The final chapter, Chapter 6, turns to practices of contention and complaint as sites of engagement with state health reforms, particularly in spaces marked off for community decision making at the local level. It ethnographically examines how residents of Machacamarca engaged in public speechmaking to complain about inadequate services, funding shortages, and unfulfilled promises in community fora. I examine the complaint as a demand for obligation and accountability in the aftermath of activism—a more minor political form that operates alongside major political forms in Bolivia like the protest and the blockade. This chapter ultimately considers how, in a context in which institutional care is always already wrapped up in colonialism, we might foreground complaint, resentment, and noncollaboration as sites of moral and political possibility. Specifically, I point to the unfinishedness of decolonization, but also to its aspirational horizons.

The book concludes with a discussion of the intertwined political and health crises that unfolded in Bolivia after the completion of fieldwork, as Evo Morales was ousted from the presidency in 2019 and as the Covid-19 pandemic hit in 2020. Ending with the return of the MAS through the election of Luis Arce in late 2020, I ask what possibilities for decolonization, accountability, and contention are still unfolding in Bolivia.

1 THE BUREAUCRATIC POLITICS OF GOOD LIVING

Health Policy in the Morales Era

IN LATE 2014, I ATTENDED a roundtable on traditional healing at the offices of the Spanish Agency for International Development Cooperation (*Agencia Española de Cooperación Internacional para el Desarrollo,* AECID) near the city center of La Paz. Fluorescent lighting lit up the bright white room, where participants gathered in chairs organized in a u-shape around the projector screen at the front of the room. The meeting brought together the Vice-Minister of Traditional Medicine and Interculturality, several of his staff members, the traditional medicine representative from the La Paz Departmental Health Service, a few representatives from traditional healer unions, and representatives from several NGOs that worked to support state policy on traditional medicine. The stated goal of the meeting was to discuss progress made thus far on implementing intercultural health policies as well as ongoing challenges; they would also discuss how the different organizations present that day could coordinate better with one another.

A vice-ministry staff member named Alonzo had been tasked with giving the opening presentation on progress made in implementing health policies pertaining to interculturality and traditional medicine.

As he was setting up the PowerPoint on the projector screen at the front of the room, several audience members began conversing.

Herculiano, an elderly Aymara man, was the head of the La Paz Departmental Federation of Ancestral Traditional Naturista Doctors, one of the major healing unions to operate in the region. He began expressing his frustration at having to attend yet another policy planning meeting:

> We have attended so many events and workshops. There's a lot of talk, but no one's doing anything. Some say that the SAFCI is doing things, but I don't know. Traditional medicine continues to be clandestine. I am sorry to say this. The [nonprofit] cooperative agencies are surely doing some things, but in other departments like Potosí and Sucre, not so much here in La Paz. I would be really grateful if we could actually start something.

Alonzo listened and nodded as Herculiano spoke. He acknowledged the healer's arguments and then redirected them: "We have to take into account the concerns of the representatives of traditional medicine. The *hermano*[1] says that there's only theory but not practice. But this is why we are doing this roundtable. Health programs are always elaborated based on the demands of the most vulnerable Indigenous populations."

Then, Alberto Camaqui,[2] the Vice-Minister of Traditional Medicine and Interculturality, joined the conversation. A middle-aged Aymara healer, he had been appointed to the position about a year before I began my research. He wore the leather jacket and fedora typical of rural union leaders. His deep voice resonating, he pronounced, "We are discussing policies of the Ministry of Health. But to be honest, if it weren't for the cooperative agencies, we would not be able to have intercultural medicine programs. If we don't work together, there will be many weaknesses in the system."

As the meeting progressed, Alonzo continued to attempt to bring the conversation back to the importance of state policies. As the conversation died down and he began his presentation, he pulled up a slide that discussed policies that the state had enacted. Referencing the debate from a few minutes earlier, Alonzo insisted, "Laws like the Law of Traditional and Ancestral Medicine are witness to how traditional healers have become political actors. This reflects what is in the Constitution about the rights of Indigenous Peasant and First Peoples. Although we have been critical of the Ministry of Health, it's easier to enact change when there are policies in place."

As I attended numerous roundtables and policy planning meetings in the city of La Paz, I often listened to preoccupations and debates about the disjuncture between "just talk" and "doing something." For Alonzo, the act of gathering itself was a site where national policy was being upheld; officials were inviting participation and elaborating interventions "based on the demands of the most vulnerable Indigenous populations." Yet for many of the participants that day, meetings were not enough: meetings did not always lead to resources being distributed or programs being supported.

While conducting research for this book, I often heard a range of comments about the limitations of health reform in Bolivia. Acquaintances who were middle- or upper-class Bolivians often emphasized to me that Evo Morales "had done nothing" for health care—a discourse that was sometimes echoed by conservative politicians and in the local media. Very often, however, these sources could not name the health laws and policies the MAS had already enacted.[3] In contrast, a different perspective emerged among those who were the primary recipients of national health policy interventions, including Indigenous traditional healers, midwives, and patients. Moments like Herculiano's complaints during the ministry meeting highlighted how many people also had aspirations for state-led decolonization, hoping it might deliver on its promises of dignified, pluralistic, and accessible care. Yet they expressed frustration as the state was seemingly unable to bring this project to fruition. They pointed to challenges around limited funding and uneven reliance on NGOs to help implement policies, as well as generally curtailed forms of implementation. The Morales administration, I suggest, did enact key steps in transforming health services for Indigenous patients within a rubric of warm care—but many policy recipients hoped that these reforms might go further.

Echoing my interlocutors who highlighted a mismatch between "just talk" and "actually doing something," scholars working in Bolivia have analyzed how the MAS's radical rhetoric and public performances did not always translate into corresponding actions on the ground.[4] Many have argued that the more limited or fragmentary version of policies put into practice reflect how, as the MAS took over dominant governing apparatuses, it shifted from a strategy of active revolution to a project of reconciliation and transformation (McNelly 2023)—one that still enacted changes, but largely within the confines of a liberal settler state system (Postero 2017). As David Mosse (2004) reminds us, moreover, disjunctures between policy design and implementation are also exceedingly common—and may even be a condition of policy itself. For him, the elements needed to mobilize political support and alliances to craft policy are different from the relationships, translations, and compromises needed to enact policy in practice. Policy, Tess Lea (2020) suggests, is at once unruly, messy, and profoundly self-replicating, haunted by past configurations that make it a difficult medium for radical transformation.

Building on these conversations, in this chapter I examine how colonial biopolitics[5] remained a durable—if not totalizing or inevitable—underpinning for state health policies across administrations. Taking a genealogical approach, I situate Morales-era health reforms against a historical backdrop of Bolivian state health care policies geared toward rural Indigenous and campesino populations, beginning with the National Revolution of 1952. I show how, despite Morales-era goals of rupturing with the past and articulating what many described as a "new way of thinking, feeling, and doing health," reforms often folded back into entrenched modes of intervention.

At the same time, taking up Choctaw anthropologist Valerie Lambert's (2022) call to be attentive to the agency that Indigenous bureaucrats assert when working within dominant state institutions, I examine how and on what terms health policymakers were able to invoke decolonial projects. I show how, especially in public-facing venues and documents, MAS bureaucrats articulated what they envisioned for a decolonized health care system. In educational documents that accompanied formal laws, as well as in interviews with me, poli-cymakers invoked Indigenous relational ethics and paradigms of well-being as the basis for a new health care system, one that would break with past colonial and capitalist formations. Across these sites, poli-cymakers sought to solidify the MAS's platform for a wider audience—but also engaged in their own ethical experimentation and theorizing about what a radically transformed health care system might entail. Yet as the larger structural transformations that many policymakers envisioned proved challenging to implement with limited funding, re-forms often shifted to a more curtailed project of emphasizing affective warmth and cultural inclusion for Indigenous patients. If decoloni-zation was at its core a proposal for structural undoing, in practice, state officials, institutions, and apparatuses also struggled to hold the tensions and disruptions such an undoing might entail. Everyday bu-reaucratic documents, practices, and infrastructures often focused more narrowly on fixing individual patient and provider behaviors, all while emphasizing the importance of being more attentive and of-fering warmth and cultural inclusion. As I show, this modality of care also reinscribed long-standing approaches to regulating Indigenous bodies and populations, often deflecting from historical and struc-tural underpinnings of illness to locate pathology within Indigenous patients themselves.

To trace these processes of uneven reinscription, this chapter takes a historical and genealogical approach. Beginning with health reforms after the 1952 national revolution, I trace how biopolitical projects of regulating Indigenous knowledges, practices, and bodies in the name of health were threaded through twentieth-century Bolivian policies. I show how across shifts in administration, particular ideas about care and intervening in Indigenous bodies and relations remained espe-cially sticky—and continued to be so even within the Morales admin-istration's decolonial projects. I turn to how Morales administration officials worked to coordinate policy implementation given resource constraints, as well as how ultimately they flattened ideas about engag-ing plural worlds through their emphasis on warm care.

DEVELOPING THE HEALTH OF THE MODERN NATION

In Bolivia, the establishment of state biomedical clinics to serve rural Indigenous patients has a relatively recent history. Occasional, incipient efforts in the early twentieth century to extend biomedical care into rural regions were uneven, often contingent on aid programs from the United States, like the Rockefeller Foundation and the Cooperative Inter-American Public Health Service (*Servicio Cooperativo Interamericano de Salud Pública*, SCISP) beginning in the 1940s (Pacino 2013; 2015; Zulawski 2007). In rural mining centers, some mining companies also provided health care to their employees (Mendizabal Lozano 2002). Many health care services—taking the form of charity hospitals and later, private clinics—were concentrated in Bolivia's larger cities (Zulawski 2007). It was not until after the National Revolution of 1952 that health care for all Bolivians was considered a responsibility of the state (Pacino 2013; Zulawski 2007). It is at this point that I begin my historical account.

Launched by a coalition of rural miners, urban workers, students, and others, the National Revolution of 1952 was the second major anti-oligarchic revolution in Latin America (following the Mexican Revolution in 1910) and marked a significant turning point in Bolivia. Upon assuming power, the Nationalist Revolutionary Movement (*Movimiento Nacionalista Revolucionario*, MNR) party nationalized the mining industry and formally put an end to large hacienda holdings in rural areas and redistributed land to *campesinos* (peasants) who worked it. It also established voting rights for women and Indigenous peoples, who had previously been denied access to full citizenship in Bolivia.[6] As historians have shown, these progressive reforms were also tied to a developmentalist project of modernizing the nation and forging a new national identity around shared *mestizaje* (racial and cultural mixture). While mestizaje had long been central to nation-state-building projects in a variety of Latin American contexts,[7] it became central to Bolivian national political discourse primarily after the 1952 revolution, precisely with the idea that it would bridge rural-urban divides and bring those who had been excluded from the nation-state into it. Bolivian national discourses of mestizaje emphasized all Bolivians' distant but shared Indigenous ancestry (Sanjinés 2004; Molina 2021). Discourses also simultaneously emphasized the need for contemporary Indigenous peoples to assimilate into whiteness—what Silvia Rivera Cusicanqui (1984; 2010) has called "colonial Andean mestizaje." As she argues, "The idea of mestizaje put forward by the MNR . . . entailed a unilateral joining [of] the Western values, language, and modes of thought . . . and excluded any form of multiculturalism or multilingualism" (1984, 129, my translation). As elsewhere in the Andes, ideologies of mestizaje centered the notion that Indigenous peoples, by adopting the language, modes of dress, and education of dominant society would shed their indigeneity and become more mestizo (de la Cadena 2000).

Alongside education, health care became a central mechanism of the project to improve and integrate the countryside into the "modern" mestizo nation post-1952. As historian Nicole Pacino (2013; 2015) describes, under the MNR, new health programs centered on vaccination, nutrition, hygiene, and maternal-infant health, as well as the construction of new health infrastructures like sanitary posts and maternal health dispensaries. These programs were simultaneously framed as a benevolent project of state care and a project of modernizing rural Indians by inculcating them with a "sanitary consciousness" (Pacino 2013, 35). Bolivian reforms mirrored health and development projects across the globe in the mid-twentieth century that positioned broad-based acceptance of biomedicine as central to progress and modernity—and tied the health of the individual to the health of the nation (Street 2014).

Many of the MNR's health initiatives were enacted as part of a joint effort with the SCISP, a United States government aid program that had been working in Bolivia since the 1940s (Pacino 2013; 2015). After the revolution, the U.S. government continued to funnel considerable aid to the MNR because it saw it as more moderate than other left governments in the region, and it wanted to prevent the rise of elements further to the left within the party during the Cold War (Siekmeier 2011; Young 2013). SCISP officials lent funding and logistical support, but also shared many Bolivian officials' concerns that Indigenous cultural practices were to blame for contagion. MNR and SCISP officials alike targeted Indigenous "customs" broadly for sanitary reform—but these concerns congealed, especially, around parenting practices and childbirth. Officials blamed Indigenous women for Bolivia's high infant mortality rates, which they argued were impeding Bolivia's progress as a nation and its ability to produce the next generation of healthy Bolivians. Pro-natalist rural health interventions emphasized the importance of clinical births, assisted by a biomedical professional, and encouraged women to reject home-birthing. Health center programs and new "mothers' clubs" also taught women about hygiene and nutrition in an effort to change domestic habits (Gallien 2015; Kimball 2020; Pacino 2015).

Linkages between medicine, race, and nation extended into later governments, even as they were articulated in new ways. In 1964, a military coup d'état overthrew the MNR-led government. The next decades fluctuated between rule by military juntas and by democratically elected governments. Right-wing military regimes frequently operated with substantial support from the U.S. government, in both the form of military aid and health and development aid, mainly via the Alliance for Progress and the United States Agency for International Development (USAID). As others studying Cold War politics in Latin America have noted, U.S. military aid and development aid to repressive dictatorships were often closely linked, as U.S. officials positioned development aid as a means to pacify populations and address the conditions of poverty, thereby preventing (or so they thought) people from turning to communism (Field 2014; Geidel 2010; Siekmeier 2011).

As before, Bolivian health policymakers collaborated closely with United States aid programs to target what they deemed to be life-threatening Indigenous "customs" and domestic practices. Yet in a shift from an earlier emphasis on pro-natalism, global aid agencies were increasingly embracing projects of family planning to limit Indigenous reproduction—a project that the Bolivian state at various points adopted and then distanced itself from (Gallien 2015; Geidel 2010; Kimball 2020). Strategies for addressing the threats presumably posed by Indigenous culture also shifted, as health programs began mobilizing community members to sustain the expansion of biomedicine in the countryside. In the global development world, community participation was used on both the left and the right, emerging as a response to the failures of top-down planning (Immerwahr 2015). For example, in 1973 the military regime of Hugo Banzer initiated a national *parto limpio* (clean birth) program to train Indigenous *parteras* (midwives) in basic biomedical techniques (Gallien 2015). USAID also later initiated projects to recruit local "community health promoters" to educate their neighbors in maternal-infant health, nutrition, infectious disease control, and environmental sanitation (Bastien 1990; Gallien 2015).

The main goal of these various programs was not to recognize "traditional" knowledges on their own terms, but to mobilize local residents to bring more people into the biomedical system. Policymakers expressed concerns that Indigenous peoples were not using available health services and blamed Indigenous culture for health center avoidance. Yet it was also during this time that Indigenous activists mobilized to push back against dictatorial regimes and demand greater recognition of their knowledge on its own terms. The practice of traditional medicine had been formally criminalized in Bolivia since the early twentieth century, but beginning in the 1960s and 1970s, Aymara and Quechua healers based in the Andes began actively organizing for decriminalization—many in connection with a broader Indigenous militant and intellectual movement known as Katarismo that sought to bridge class struggle with Indian ethnic struggle (Álvarez Quispe and Loza 2014; Burman 2017). Walter Álvarez Quispe, a Kallawaya healer and biomedical doctor, described in a later published interview that he and others had grown frustrated with dialogues organized by the Bolivian state and the Jesuit Church that proposed limited institutional integration for healers. Instead, he ended up organizing for decriminalization as health secretary for the Syndical Confederation of Rural Workers of Bolivia (*Confederación Sindical Única de Trabajadores Campesinos de Bolivia*, CSUTCB), a peasant union that had emerged out of the Katarista movement as an alternative to state-sponsored peasant unions (Álvarez Quispe and Loza 2014). Anders Burman likewise notes that ritual healers involved in the CSUTCB played a key role in revitalizing ancestral knowledge, performing rituals, and theorizing the sickness of colonial modernity. Therefore, they centrally "contributed to the 'indianization' of the discourse and politics of the rural syndicate" (2017, 55).

FROM SOCIAL MEDICINE TO NEOLIBERAL MULTICULTURALISM

As the Carter administration in the United States sought to reverse the government's agenda of supporting Latin American dictators, it pressured Bolivia to undertake a regulated "democratic opening" at the end of the 1970s. After several years of power struggle between Bolivia's military leaders—who resisted a democratic transition—Hernán Siles Zuazo was elected president of Bolivia by a wide margin in 1982 (Klein 2011).

Siles Zuazo's administration, associated with the left wing of the MNR, positioned itself as closely aligned with the progressive health goals of the 1978 Alma Ata Accords and the paradigm of social medicine more broadly (Torres-Goitia 2010; Torres-Goitia and Burgoa 2015). Following the tenets of the Latin American Social Medicine movement, Bolivian policymakers turned to addressing health in relation to broader social and economic determinants. New initiatives such as the Integral Program of Health Area Services (*Programa Integral de Atención de Áreas de Salud*, PIAAS) established "health areas" in the countryside, each under the charge of a doctor and a community health team that would engage in primary care and preventative health work (Torres-Goitia 2010; Torres-Goitia and Burgoa 2015).

In 1984, in response to pressures from traditional healing activists like those organizing through the CSUTCB, as well as shifting approaches to traditional medicine within the WHO, the Bolivian legislature also decriminalized the practice of traditional medicine, becoming the first country in Latin America to formally do so. It also formalized the status of the Bolivian Society for Traditional and Ancestral Medicine (*Sociedad Boliviana de Medicina Tradicional*, SOBOMETRA) as the nation's official institution for the research, training, and advocacy of healing (Babis 2014; Campos Navarro 1997; Loza 2008; Nigenda et al. 2001). Yet while decriminalization was an important step that addressed a longtime demand of healing activists, Bolivian officials largely continued their predecessors' policies of mobilizing healers as a local resource to facilitate the practice of biomedicine in rural areas. As Dr. Javier Torres-Goitia, minister of health at the time, described a project for bringing Kallawaya healers into PIAAS health teams, "We established a beneficial exchange. [The Kallawaya healers] helped us understand the expression of Indigenous psychology to orient our work, and they received with enthusiasm the modern scientific knowledge that the PIAAS doctors were able to transmit to them" (Torres-Goitia and Burgoa 2015, 101, my translation).

At the same time, efforts to transform the health care system remained patchwork, as there was little funding to carry out projects like the PIAAS (Torres-Goitia 2010). President Siles Zuazo faced a tanking economy and international debt crisis when he came into office, and hyperinflation increased dramatically over his brief tenure (Klein 2011). He agreed to hold early elections for a new president in 1985, and his successor, President Victor Paz Estenssoro, almost immediately instated a program of neoliberal shock therapy—what became known as the "New Economic Plan." Under the guidance of economic advisors from the United States, the Bolivian government undertook currency devaluation, free market reforms, and radical cuts to state spending in health, education, and other public services. If these reforms succeeded in curtailing hyperinflation, they also came at an enormous social cost. They were met with frequent protest, as unemployment and food prices soared and social services were cut (Bailey and Knutsen 1987; Conaghan, Malloy, and Abugattas 1990; Klein 2011; Young 2013).

Neoliberal structural adjustment policies continued into the 1990s and early 2000s under subsequent administrations, often in line with conditions set out by International Monetary Fund (IMF) loans. Yet, as political scientist Christina Ewig (2010) notes, reforms beginning in the mid-1990s in Latin America—what she calls "second-wave neoliberalism"—took a different form from the shock therapy of the earlier first wave. Responding to widespread criticism of neoliberal shock therapy's severe effects on marginalized members of society, reformers paired ongoing privatization, free market policies, and state decentralization with limited social programs. The World Bank, for example, suggested that economic growth and streamlining government spending on the health sector would ultimately improve the health of the poor (Foley 2010; Keshavjee 2014). In Bolivia, the neoliberal administration of President Sánchez de Lozada enacted multiple health reforms. On the one hand, it established the new Universal Maternal and Child Insurance (*Seguro Universal Materno Infantil,* SUMI) that provided health care free of cost for maternal and child care (Kimball 2020). At the same time, echoing other forms of "neoliberal governmentality" (Gupta and Sharma 2006), the state increasingly turned to an influx of NGOs to help provide health care services under an increasingly decentralizing state.

Simultaneously, in the early 1990s, a growing Indigenous rights movement in Bolivia, as well as around the globe, pushed the state to move away from tactics of assimilation that had shaped policy since 1952 toward a policy of rights and recognition. For the first time recognizing Bolivia's "multicultural" character, policies shifted to support cultural and territorial rights for Indigenous peoples, albeit on limited terms. New policies supported popular participation in local policies (Postero 2007; Regalsky 2005) as well as intercultural education (Gustafson 2009b) and health care. For example, the new SUMI law called for intercultural maternal health care "to be adapted to the practices, customs, languages, and dialects of indigenous, campesino, and original peoples" (cited in Kimball 2020, 193). Also in 2002, in an agreement developed with the CSUTCB, state officials developed a plan to credential traditional healers to work in public hospitals and clinics. However, this project was never implemented because of President Sánchez de Lozada's ouster from office (Kimball 2020; Loza 2008).

As Nancy Postero (2007) argues, while shifts in national policy were arguably a significant shift away from the assimilationist state and opened up new avenues for political claims-making, many were dissatisfied with the limits of these reforms. Amid ongoing economic

marginalization caused by neoliberal austerity measures, social movements expressed frustration at both the lack of economic mobility and
the insufficiency of state cultural recognition paradigms. During Sánchez de Lozada's second term, in 2003—in what would later become
known as the Gas War—numerous social movements joined protests
in El Alto and other major Bolivian cities to protest the proposal of a
gas pipeline to Chile, tying it to broader problems with privatization
and lack of redistribution of wealth. Sánchez de Lozada authorized the
military to use force to control the protests. The military killed eighty
civilians, including many children and bystanders. In the aftermath,
Sánchez de Lozada resigned and fled to the United States (where he
remains to this day). He was succeeded by several interim governments before new elections were held in 2005 and Evo Morales won
by a landslide.[8]

A NEW WAY OF DOING HEALTH?

Evo Morales, an Aymara campesino originally from the highland
region of Oruro, later migrated to the lowland Chapare region with
his family to grow coca. He began his social movement work through
the agricultural union representing coca growers in the region. What
later became the MAS emerged from efforts to develop an electoral
arm of the Six Federations of the Tropics of Cochabamba. Early in his
political career, Morales campaigned to demand an end to U.S.-backed
coca-eradication policies, which relied on violent strategies of military
suppression. The MAS also increasingly allied itself with other movements, gaining national visibility and momentum after its participation in protests against the privatization of the municipal water supply
in Cochabamba in 2000 (Farthing and Kohl 2014; Grisaffi 2019). Many
commentators have attributed Morales's momentous win in the 2005
presidential elections to the coalition work that he and the MAS undertook bridging multiple political sectors, including workers' unions,
Indigenous rights organizations, and popular neighborhood associations, as well as left-leaning members of the middle class, particularly
in the wake of massive mobilizations against neoliberal privatization

and structural adjustment measures. The Morales administration's broad-based agenda promised an end to neoliberal austerity measures and a turn to state investment in redistributive social programs. It also promised the deepening of Indigenous cultural and territorial rights that would go beyond the limited forms of multicultural recognition that had been state policy since the early 1990s (Goodale 2019; Postero 2017).

Upon assuming office, the Morales administration undertook sweeping reforms, including the convening of a new constitutional assembly that would ultimately rewrite the national constitution and "re-found" Bolivia as a plurinational state. On the one hand, the plurinational state would deepen cultural and territorial rights for Bolivia's thirty-six officially recognized Indigenous nations, ostensibly moving beyond superficial forms of multicultural recognition. At the same time, the state would take on a more central role in investing in social programs and ensuring the redistribution of resources.[9] Although the MAS never fully embraced socialism (despite what the party name would indicate), the Morales administration did partially nationalize some industries and invest in social spending, much of which went to public infrastructure projects (for example, roads, hospitals, satellite networks) and conditional cash payments (such as for the elderly, pregnant women, and schoolchildren) (Postero 2017; Gustafson 2020). Bringing these multiple paradigms—Indigenous rights and state-led redistribution—together, the Morales administration brought forward a national development plan that put forward a vision of a decolonized state, one that centered a broadly Indigenous relational ethics of *Vivir Bien* (good living) (Ministerio de Planificación del Desarollo 2007). Vivir Bien offered an ethical paradigm for state policy to foreground both a plurality of ways of being but also emphasize equality, reciprocity, and community (as opposed to extractive colonial-capitalist models, under which people did not live well) (Schavelzón 2012). These proposals provided an overarching guide for reforms in numerous areas, including health care.

Upon taking office in 2006, Evo Morales appointed Dr. Nila Heredia—a mestiza physician, social medicine advocate, and political activist who had been imprisoned during the military dictatorship—as Minister of Health and Sports. With the goal of drafting policy to reshape the health care system, Dr. Heredia put together a multidisciplinary team of people (including doctors, sociologists, and public health experts) who had prior experiences with rural and community-based health care. These included a number who had worked for the PIAAS in the 1980s as well as many who had worked for NGOs during the neoliberal years. In addition to bringing in people who had prior experience in rural and community health, the team also held public assemblies in each of the nine departments in Bolivia with biomedical practitioners, traditional healers, and civil society actors in advance of incorporating language on health care into the national constitution (Bernstein 2017; Johnson 2010).

The result was a new national policy, the Family, Community, and Intercultural Health Law (*Salud Familiar Comunitaria e Intercultural,* or SAFCI)—under development since 2006 but formally signed into law in 2008 (Johnson 2010). The policy offered a paradigm of care for the public state-run health care system, particularly at the primary care level. The SAFCI proposed changes in *gestión* (health care management, administration) to foreground community decision making in local health care measures. Simultaneously, changes addressing *atención* (care, treatment) proposed a more expansive form of care that would take into account socioeconomic and cultural dimensions of patients' experiences. The latter also included what policymakers called *interculturalidad* (interculturality)—the incorporation of biomedical and traditional medical practices on equal footing (Ministerio de Salud y Deportes 2008). In short, the goal was to build a preventative and community-based model of primary care (inspired by other social medicine models in the region) while also making room for a plurality of medical knowledges and ontologies to operate within this system.

Following on the heels of this law, in 2013 the Law of Traditional and Ancestral Medicine further formalized the status of traditional healers and their integration within the national health care system, expanding on the provisions for interculturality included in the SAFCI (Asamblea Legislativa Plurinacional de Bolivia 2013a). Developed with the active participation of healing unions, it created a national registry and unified system for credentialing healers—a longtime demand of traditional healer unions and federations in Bolivia, who positioned credentials as a key source of legitimacy given the fact that the practice of traditional medicine had been criminalized in Bolivia until 1984.

These two new laws, positioned as central mechanisms for decolonizing health care, worked in tandem with other projects to extend state care. One major item on the Ministry of Health's agenda was the implementation of a universal health care system, but it had difficulty getting off the ground (Johnson 2010). Bolivia's health care system was fragmented between a private sector (paid out of pocket), employer insurance-based clinics (known as *cajas*), and a public system (Ledo and Soria 2011). The goal of universal health care was to make the public system free for patients. However, the project struggled with entrenched opposition from *cajas* and doctors' unions, as well as problems with ongoing infrastructural shortages. The Morales administration did eventually enact a state-run option (known as the Single Health System) for those without other insurance in early 2019, some months before Evo Morales was ousted from office (Asamblea Legislativa Plurinacional de Bolivia 2019). Its implementation has been patchwork—although President Luís Arce, elected in 2020, stated that he would make it a priority to revitalize the program (Booth 2020). For most of my research period, most public services were offered at a relatively low cost, and certain groups (children under five, pregnant and postpartum women, the elderly, and the disabled) received care for free, expanding and consolidating the SUMI program begun under Sánchez de Lozada in the 1990s. A new program (called the Bono Juana Azurduy) also provided conditional cash payments for pregnant and postpartum women.

Both the making and implementation of policy were marked by numerous tensions, challenges, and points of unevenness. One challenge, especially in the early years of Morales's presidency, was racist backlash and entrenched opposition to his policies, especially among the wealthy in the lowland regions of Santa Cruz, Beni, and Pando (known as the Media Luna region). Engaged in a separatist movement for regional autonomy, they also sought to block numerous Morales administration reforms (Fabricant 2009; Goodale 2019). These conflicts had reverberating effects for health care as well. As Brian Johnson (2010) describes, departmental governors in the Media Luna region initially discouraged cooperation with the SAFCI policy because they saw it as too closely tied to the MAS. Organizations like the College of Physicians (that organized all doctors in the country) also proclaimed opposition to the policy because they saw it as opening the path for community representatives to exert too much control over their activities (Johnson 2010). In later years, some of this opposition calmed, particularly as the MAS, perhaps out of political necessity, also made concessions to Media Luna elites (much to the discontentment of some of its more progressive base). The College of Physicians continued to protest numerous other policies as infringing on their autonomy of practice, including, in 2019, efforts to move toward universal health care.

Yet different sets of tensions also started to emerge among those who largely supported the MAS's health reforms. As I show in the pages that follow, as policymakers weighed what decolonization of the health care system might entail, they confronted the limitations of working through a system forged through colonialism—where infrastructures had already been built around regulating Indigenous life, and where unequal national and global resource flows continued to constrain funding for new projects. In turn, many policy recipients had hopes for state-led reform, but expressed frustration that new policies were not always being implemented as promised.

INDIGENOUS TECHNOLOGIES OF POWER

One weekday evening in 2014, I joined Alonzo, the staffer from the Vice-Ministry of Traditional Medicine and Interculturality who gave the presentation at the roundtable, for tea in the city center of La Paz. He had left his office late—at nearly 8 p.m.—and looked tired and harried when he met me at the obelisk statue on the city's main boulevard. Yet he shook my hand warmly, greeting me with his customary enthusiasm, as he asked me where we should go that evening. When we had first met a year before, Alonzo had expressed considerable interest in my research, pronouncing that he would tell me all there was to know about traditional medicine and healing. Like many people I met over the course of my field research, he equated my study of health policies with a wider interest in traditional medicine—a topic that fell more in line with what many people imagined anthropologists studied. Yet the doctor's interest in the traditional was also part of his own project of self-discovery—one that profoundly shaped the ways he approached work at the vice-ministry. Initially trained as a dentist, he was completing his master's degree in sociology at the Public University of El Alto through part-time study. He researched traditional medicine for his thesis, and on the weekends, he played in an Andean folk music group. Although he had not grown up speaking Aymara, he was working toward learning the language of his parents and grandparents.

We decided that evening to walk to a small café near the obelisk, pushing our way through the throng of commuters lining up for rides on the mini-buses that would take them back home to El Alto. The café itself was relatively empty, the regular hour for afternoon tea having come and gone. As we sat down, we each ordered anise tea and a pastry, and I pulled out a hard copy of the proposal for what was at the time my doctoral dissertation. We had previously discussed my bringing it so that he could offer his thoughts and feedback. He now looked over the short document that included a bullet-point outline and brief discussion of my tentative conceptual framings concerning the state, biopolitics, and well-being. As he read along the page, he shook his head. "No, no," he insisted. "This doesn't reflect our process of change." He began scribbling an alternative outline for my proposal on the back of the print-out. I have translated his outline below:

1. Bolivian Health System (as it currently exists):
   Elements:
   - Individual
   - Colonizing
   - Political

- Ideological
- Hegemonic
- Liberal/Neoliberal

2. Indigenous Health System:
   Elements:
   - Communitarian
   - Cosmological
   - Ancestral
   - Historical

3. Proposal for a New Paradigm:
   A health care system that is:
   Elements:
   - Intercultural
   - Integral
   - Communitarian
   - Universal[10]

Alonzo was an enthusiastic supporter of the MAS—and like many bureaucrats I interviewed, he expressed optimism that the state, while still in a process of transformation, could operate as a meaningful vehicle for social change.[11] Bolivian health policymakers came from a range of backgrounds: some of them, like Alonzo, identified as Aymara or as Indigenous, while others positioned themselves as mestizo or as unmarked in their identities. Many had prior experience working on health policy projects or in the NGO world. While they sometimes disagreed about precise approaches, most were hopeful about the project of enacting change as laid out by the MAS platform.

The outline that Alonzo provided closely echoed how many state officials described the goals of health care reform, as well as many of the framings that could be found in informational documents produced by the Ministry of Health. In rewriting my outline for me, Alonzo hoped that my work might illuminate for an international audience what the Morales administration was working to achieve. But it was also one of many instances when, over the course of interviews and conversations, health policymakers would theorize what the decolonization of the Bolivian health care system would entail. Like Alonzo, many emphasized the centrality of engaging Indigenous cosmologies and understandings of health as a guide for a reimagined health care system. In Alonzo's outline, the Indigenous health system (one that was "communitarian, cosmological, ancestral, historical") could lead into a new paradigm for health care (that would be "intercultural, integral, communitarian, universal"). Policymakers did not simply seek to include Indigenous traditional medicines within the health care system (although doing so was part of policy reforms). Rather, they sought to completely reframe how institutions approached the question of health and administered care.

Ramón, another bureaucrat working at the Ministry of Health, described this process as working to create "Indigenous technologies of power." A tall, energetic sociologist with black hair tied back in a ponytail and an earring in one of his lobes, he worked as head of the unit on health administration for the ministry. On one of our first meetings, I had walked into his office at the tail end of his lunch break and found him leaning back in his office chair reading a Spanish translation of Michel Foucault's *The Birth of the Clinic* (1994). Several other books by Foucault were stacked on his desk. After I greeted him, I asked him what he thought of the books, mentioning that I had also had to read many of the same works for my courses. "They are good," replied Ramón. "This is what we are trying to do—create Indigenous technologies of power."

Like Alonzo and Ramón, state bureaucrats working in the Morales administration often pondered, thought out loud about, and debated what it might mean to imagine a radically transformed health care system. They often drew from numerous intellectual genealogies and projects, bringing together the writings of European philosophers (such as Foucault, Marx, Hardt, and Negri) with those of decolonial theory, both from abroad (for example, Fanon, Dussel) and from Bolivia (for example, Reinaga, Patzi, Huanacuni, and others). I suggest that these ponderings constituted a central form of ethical experimentation, in which policymakers could also articulate and imagine possibilities for health care otherwise. They engaged in these forms of experimentation especially during interviews and conversations with me, knowing that doing so was a way to clarify their goals for an international and academic audience. They also did so in the production of didactic and framing documents that accompanied national laws and were geared toward explaining new policies to administrators, health officials, biomedical providers, and others. In articulating their project for others, they sought to solidify their vision of a transformed health care. Many Bolivian policy reformers I interviewed focused their efforts on challenging Eurocentric epistemologies and ontologies of health, understanding struggles over knowledge, care, and praxis in medicine to also be struggles against colonial and capitalist processes (see Abadía-Barrero 2022). As Lambert (2022) has argued, working to transform political and legal concepts has also been a way for Indigenous bureaucrats to work to shift the parameters of the settler state from within. Broadly allied MAS bureaucrats engaged with decolonial theory to conceptually reimagine how entrenched state and biopolitical apparatuses might operate (see also Bohrt 2019).

Much like Ramón, many bureaucrats I interviewed were not interested in shedding biopolitical apparatuses all together. Rather, the goal was to remake the biopolitical from an Indigenous standpoint. Elaborating on what he meant by "Indigenous technologies of power," Ramón described to me how it might provide a basis for reimagining strategies for health care. He explained,

> The SAFCI is not just dedicated to [the health of] man. That is, it's not, say, anthropocentric. When we speak, for example, of our concept of "integrality," we are talking about the health of man with all beings, that is, with the *Madre Tierra* [Mother Earth], with the cosmos. So that's a difference with PHC [Primary Health Care]. It's a new form of understanding health that man is in equilibrium with nature, with Mother Earth. Now, we are still missing a lot of the instruments to put this [framework] into practice—we are still speaking of the conceptual.

In redefining health, Ramón reframed social medicine's emphasis on primary health care provision to center Indigenous ontological relations with earth beings. His redefinition of health foregrounded the centrality of relations with other-than-human entities like the Madre Tierra (a loose Spanish translation of the Aymara word *Pachamama*). His invocation of the Madre Tierra might be understood as what Marisol de la Cadena (2010; 2015) has described as an Indigenous cosmopolitics, in which engaging with earth beings as political actors can disrupt the Eurocentric and normative foundations of politics itself (see also Escobar 2020; Blaser 2009). For Ramón and many other officials, bringing in relations with other-than-humans was a starting point not just for reimagining politics, but for challenging the very terms of "health" itself. Many state bureaucrats I interviewed critiqued what they described as the pervasiveness of *asistencialismo* (biomedical intervention focused primarily on treatment of the biological body) in Bolivian health care settings. Invoking the state's wider promise to sustain Vivir Bien, they called for a more holistic conception of health that incorporated primary and preventative care, as well as attention to social and environmental contexts.

These framings also figured centrally in numerous didactic and guiding documents that the Ministry of Health issued. While the language of the laws signed by the president was often fairly cut and dried, accompanying documents designed to provide guidance to administrators, local health officials, and biomedical providers often articulated a more expansive redefinition of health. For example, one of the key guides for the SAFCI policy traced the colonial and capitalist definitions of health care and put forward a new paradigm of health, echoing Ramón's definition: "In this context health is defined as a process of bio-psycho-social, cultural, and spiritual equilibrium and harmony of the person with their surroundings, which implicates the family, the community, and nature" (Ministerio de Salud y Deportes 2008, 20, my translation).

As Brian Johnson (2010) notes, two key genealogies of activist thought shaped discussions of health care reform under the MAS: social medicine activism and activism oriented around sustaining traditional medicine and interculturality. Invoking frameworks put forward by the hemispheric movement known as Latin American

Social Medicine (LASM), policymakers I interviewed highlighted the importance of addressing socioeconomic factors underpinning health and illness, investing in primary health care and preventative health services, and sustaining the right to health through projects like universal health care. Rooted in Marxist principles, LASM was solidified as a hemispheric movement in the 1970s, building in part on the work toward health care reform undertaken by President Salvador Allende in Chile before his death in the 1973 coup d'état. A regional association, the Latin American Association of Social Medicine, was founded in 1984 to bring together scholars and activists working on social medicine in the region (Laurens, Abadía-Barrero, and Hernández 2023).[12] Dr. Heredia explained in our interview, for example, that Bolivian health policy reforms were in part inspired by other countries that had adopted social medicine approaches, including Cuba, Venezuela, and especially Brazil. The Morales administration also struck accords with Cuba, inviting Cuban medical humanitarian brigades to provide medical care in Bolivia; numerous Bolivians, in turn, were able to go study medicine in Cuba and return to practice in Bolivia (Bernstein 2013).

Yet while they drew from many principles of social medicine, many officials I interviewed also insisted that a limitation of social medicine was its biomedical focus and lack of attention to Indigenous knowledges and practices of healing. Policymakers highlighted that, in a majority Indigenous country, such practices were fundamental to many people's understandings of health and thus needed to be centered in the new policies.[13] To this end, policy redefinitions of health drew from numerous activist and scholarly genealogies of reclaiming Indigenous epistemologies and ontologies in Bolivia. Perhaps most influentially, Aymara political theorist Fausto Reinaga (1940) and the Indianista-Katarista thinkers who came after him argued that the Tawatinsuyu (Incan Empire) was based in communal forms of life and well-being that offered substantive alternatives to the exploitation of capitalist systems. Building on these earlier theorizations of Aymara and Quechua communal ethics, the term *Vivir Bien* started to be popularized in policy and intellectual circles in the 1990s. At the time, the German bilateral cooperation (GTZ) commissioned a series of anthropological

studies of plural Indigenous knowledges in Bolivia; resulting publications by Aymara scholars Simón Yampara (1996; 2011), Mario Tórrez
Eguino (2012), and mestizo scholar Javier Medina (2001) put forward
Vivir Bien as a broadly Indigenous relational ethics of well-being. They
and others who have engaged the concept (Albó 2009; Huanacuni 2010;
Choquehuanca 2010) argued that Vivir Bien could operate as the basis
for a more just society, founded in reciprocity, harmony, and redistribution, in opposition to the colonial-capitalist extractivist logics of
vivir mejor ("living better").

Especially as articulated in health policy texts and by health policymakers, Vivir Bien and other implied references to Indigenous concepts of relational well-being (for example, "harmony of the person
with their surroundings," "the family, the community, and nature")
figured in broad, generalized terms. That is, policy texts did not reference the knowledges or practices of specific Indigenous nations
or communities, nor did they address differences among them. But
specificity was also not the goal. Rather, policy texts and policymakers invoked a broad conception of Indigenous *cosmovisión* (cosmol-
ogy, worldview) in binary opposition to colonial-capitalist systems
and as the basis for building an alternative to these systems. Joanne
Rappaport, in her work with Indigenous activists and intellectuals developing proposals for interculturalism in Colombia, points out that
their proposals invoke "culture" not as an ethnographic descriptor,
but rather as the basis for a "utopian political philosophy aimed at
achieving interethnic dialogue based on relations of equivalence and
at constructing a particular mode of indigenous citizenship in a plural
nation" (2005, 7). Her argument moves beyond the idea that reified notions of Indigeneity are primarily a question of strategic essentialism;
instead, her argument echoes those of others who have pointed to how
Indigenous communities also meaningfully engage in self-affirmative
essentialism (Coulthard 2014) or understand binarism to be a generative point of political engagement (Wolfe 2013). Like Rappaport, I
found that Indigenous intellectuals and bureaucrats, as well as allied
actors, frequently talked about a broad conception of Indigenous cos-
mology to create the basis of political action as well as collaboration

with health reform advocates involved with other related projects, like social medicine or community health work. That is, not all people promoting social medicine within the Ministry of Health came from a tradition of decolonial activism, but they could agree that attending to multiple kinds of relations was important, and they could agree that it was important to attend to local cultural practices. Vivir Bien, in principle, created a broad ground of shared action around health care.[14]

While drawing on broader decolonial activist proposals, health officials also built on existing paradigms for approaching Indigenous health. In developing a pluralist approach to health care, policymakers also drew considerable inspiration from other regional models of *salud intercultural* (intercultural health). Interculturality, more broadly, has been taken up in numerous Latin American policy contexts as an approach to managing cultural differences within plural societies (García 2005; Gustafson 2009b). Lucía Guerra-Reyes notes that "[a]s an applied concept, interculturality is usually operationalized in specific policies and programs as respectful and equal dialogue, identification of cultural misunderstandings, and accommodations arrived at through mutual negotiation" (2019, 14). Intercultural health—oriented around the recognition and limited incorporation of Indigenous medicines and practices into the formal health care system—has been promoted by the Pan-American Health Organization (PAHO) and taken up by numerous national governments in the region since the early and mid-2000s.[15] Bolivian health policymakers directly built from prior initiatives, compiling, for example, what they called "experiences" from NGOs that had been doing intercultural health work in the 1990s. But they also simultaneously distanced themselves from prior Bolivian initiatives as well as other models in the region by emphasizing that they were going further in creating a space for medical pluralism. Ramón put it this way:

> The WHO for example talks about cultural competency in health services. . . . But we are convinced that what they call cultural competency is just one aspect; it's not interculturality in health care. For example, in Peru, they do cultural adaptation of maternal wards. But it's a totally

utilitarian perspective. Why do you want to adapt? Why do you want to contextualize? So that people come more to your health service, to attract more people, to make the health centers more attractive.[16]

He emphasized that, in contrast, Bolivian health policies were not utilitarian attempts to encourage more people to seek care in biomedical settings but were focused on supporting and valorizing Indigenous knowledges on their own terms. Other policymakers similarly emphasized that new health policies would support the practice of Indigenous medicine on an equal footing with biomedicine. As Alonzo explained during our interview, "The articulation of two medicines [Indigenous and biomedical] is nothing more than reciprocity. It is a mutual understanding. Through interculturality, we act horizontally, where no one is above, and no one is below. Each one of us, we have our ways of thinking, but we also have respect for our beliefs."

In sum, policymakers envisioned what they often described as a "new way of thinking, feeling, and doing health" as merging tenets of social medicine (like the right to health and attention to socioeconomic determinants of health) with Indigenous ontologies of health, illness, and care. The latter included both reenvisioning how the ministry approached the question of health more broadly and creating space for a radical pluralism, where Indigenous traditional medicine and biomedicine might be treated on equal footing within the health care system. They especially articulated these new visions in interviews with me and in policy guidance documents; both spaces were essential to solidifying the MAS platform and also for policymakers themselves to ethically experiment and dwell on possibilities for a decolonized health care system.

FLATTENING THE PLURIVERSE

In early 2015, I interviewed Miguel, a Ministry of Health functionary who headed the *Mi Salud* (My Health) program, a program designed to help put the SAFCI into practice. We discussed how policymakers envisioned implementing a more expansive approach to health, and he

referenced the importance of tactics such as having doctors adminis-
ter surveys known as *carpetas familiares* (family files) to the households
in their district. He explained,

> [The doctors work] with the community via household visits, using the
> household survey. Once the survey is filled out, it allows us to identify
> health risks: personal risks, risks at the level of the family and the
> community. . . . Once we have identified the social determinants [of
> health] we can let the municipal governments and grassroots orga-
> nizations know what they are, so that they can contribute to solving
> these problems—which isn't easy, which isn't easy.

I followed up to ask what he would consider to be a social deter-
minant of health. He turned to the central example of diarrhea, a
common illness in Bolivia that he pointed out was related to lack of
potable water supply. Thus if the household surveys noted that people
did not have access to safe water supply, grassroots organizations, the
municipal government, and the health personnel could work to address it. He elaborated, "They can make it so that the water is better
quality, so that it is treated, so that there's a clean tank."

In emphasizing the centrality of clean water supply, Miguel echoed
what many social medicine advocates as well as medical anthropologists have also argued: that attending to structural and root causes
of illness, rather than blaming individual behavior, is essential for
sustaining health. Miguel drew heavily from a social determinants
of health framework, but also situated it alongside other decolonial
goals, including enacting structural transformation and centrally involving grassroots associations in local health care decisions. Yet as
Miguel also reflected, developing concrete solutions to root problems
"isn't easy." Putting in new pipes, tanks, and water treatment systems
was costly—and while the MAS had made some headway in improving
water supply in Bolivia via the *Mi Agua* (My Water) program, many municipalities remained without access to clean water.[17] Municipal governments, grassroots organizations, and biomedical providers could
identify the issue at hand but often did not have the funds to overhaul
local water and sanitation systems.

Some months after my conversation with Miguel, after I had begun working in the highland municipality of Machacamarca, I had the chance to look at the household surveys he had described. As I analyze in Chapter 5, the questions in the household surveys placed heavy emphasis on individual and household practices, such as what people ate, how many people slept to a room in a household, and what their relationship to other family members was like. The surveys positioned familial and individual behavior as the central site of risk and surveillance, moving away from the more expansive approach to addressing health inequalities promised by policymakers via the attention to social medicine and Indigenous relationality. The surveys, I suggest, ultimately reinscribed racializing tropes that had long underpinned Bolivian health care policies: that Indigenous relations and practices were themselves largely to blame for poor health outcomes.

Yet even as the surveys narrowed the focus of health intervention, state officials and nonprofit actors often emphasized that the surveys were essential for improving relations between biomedical providers and patients. They pointed to frequent distrust patients expressed toward biomedical providers, as well as the need for biomedical providers to leave the clinic to understand the health issues facing patients. The surveys, they suggested, offered a systematic way to increase contact between providers and patients.

The implementation of the household surveys reflected a wider pattern that I came to observe while conducting research on Bolivian health policy. Policymakers often identified structural underpinnings of health and illness, including concerns like clean water supply, as well as historically rooted dynamics of colonialism and capitalism. Addressing these underpinnings, however, proved to be difficult, often because of limited funding and resources (conditions that were themselves partially produced through layered dynamics of global neocolonialism and capitalism). In practice, policy interventions tended to be narrower in scope and often continued to reinscribe long-standing forms of situating Indigenous subjects as sources of pathology to be fixed and improved. Yet even as they reentrenched these forms of fixing, policymakers emphasized the centrality of being attentive, inclusive, and affectively warm toward Indigenous patients.

State bureaucrats, I argue, remained determined to improve care for Indigenous patients. But working with limited resources and within existing health apparatuses, they often found it easier to enact change within a paradigm of warm care—one that might emphasize cultural inclusion and respect but that largely maintained existing biomedical and biopolitical modes of intervention. While often bureaucratic techniques of governance—such as household data collection—socially produce indifference (Herzfeld 1993), policymakers sought to remake these apparatuses so that they were more respectful, more culturally inclusive, and more affectively warm. They positioned surveys as a way for providers to be more attentive to patients and encouraged biomedical providers to treat patients more kindly in clinical encounters. New technologies such as culturally adapted birthing rooms and medicinal plant greenhouses, along with the incorporation of Indigenous traditional midwives and healers, were likewise positioned as ways for patients to feel more included.

This focus on warmth, cultural inclusion, and kindness broke from many policymakers' focus on Indigenous cosmovisión as the basis for redefining health itself and constructing a radically pluralist system of care. Still, some policymakers reflected that Indigenous therapies also provided a model for a warmer, more attentive medical care practice. Jaime Zalles, the first Vice-Minister of Traditional Medicine and Interculturality under Evo Morales, had long been a proponent of the idea that Indigenous care practices offered more humane and attentive treatment than biomedical systems of intervention (see Zalles 1995); as Bolivian medical historian Beatriz Loza (2008) noted, under Zalles's leadership, programs largely evacuated traditional medicine of its spiritual and ontological content, instead focusing more on those aspects legible to a dominant biomedical system (see also Burman 2012). Focusing primarily on warm care, I suggest, became a way of extending respect and cultural inclusion to patients, but without fully engaging their worlds and without disrupting the existing functioning of the health care system.

As I argue throughout this book, narrowing the focus of reform to making existing health care apparatuses warmer and more inclusive did not necessarily reverse long-standing forms of structural violence—under which, as Akhil Gupta (2012) suggests, even well-meaning bureaucratic state systems create arbitrary experiences of care for intended recipients. Instead, I suggest that a shift to making bureaucratic and policy apparatuses warmer extended long-standing biopolitical modes that positioned Indigenous bodies and populations as threats to biological health, in need of targeted surveillance, regulation, and improvement. In fact, practices of health documentation and surveillance often intensified under the Morales administration, as ministry officials developed new mechanisms for keeping track of household practices, traditional healing and midwifery practices, and patient records. This reentrenchment of the biopolitical was in part an outcome of limited funding, as bureaucrats and administrators found it easier to shift interventions onto regulating individual behaviors than to addressing structural solutions, as Miguel had initially proposed. But it also reflected how racialized constructions and forms of biopolitical surveillance were baked into the very infrastructures, documents, coordinations, practices, and affects that had long been the basis of making the Bolivian health care system function. To echo Tess Lea (2020), these reproductions did not have a singular origin, but were often unevenly reinscribed and naturalized across various sites. In short, if Ramón hoped to create new "Indigenous technologies of power," existing technologies of power remained potent and largely intact, absorbing discourses about Indigenous relationality into their functioning.

It was not a contradiction for reforms to, on the one hand, intensify mechanisms of biopolitical surveillance and, on the other, extend new forms of warmth and inclusion. As I have shown throughout this chapter, over the course of Bolivian health policy history, projects of regulation and care have often gone hand in hand. Furthermore, as Indigenous Studies scholars have emphasized, liberal settler state extensions of cultural recognition, as well as moral sentiments of sympathy and repair, can often work to shore up state power and deflect from

Indigenous struggles for self-determination (Coulthard 2014; Povinelli 2002; Million 2013; Simpson 2014; 2020). As Bolivian health policies subsumed the project of decolonization to a more generalized project of warmth, they ultimately sustained the status quo.

RECRUITING INSTITUTIONS, COORDINATING POLICY

The project of warm care, I argue, also helped facilitate coordinations across a fragmentary health landscape and recruit numerous actors into a project of state reform. Warm care, in this context, could also be invoked in different ways by different institutions, but ultimately proved to be a shared common ground for intervention. One afternoon while I was conducting a lengthy interview with Ramón in his office in the Ministry of Health, our conversation was interrupted by his office phone ringing. Such interruptions were a common occurrence. Ministry of Health officials were incredibly busy, and when they graciously took the time out of their workdays to talk to me, we frequently paused the interview to accommodate phone calls and other bureaucrats knocking on the office door with urgent matters. So, when the phone rang, I knew to simply turn off my recording device and wait quietly (as Ramón said he did not mind me staying in the room). After he hung up, he turned to me and mentioned that it had been Alicia, the field director for the NGO I call GHA, on the phone. Alicia had been the one to pass me Ramón's contact information, and he knew that I had also been shadowing the NGO. He shared that Alicia had called him because GHA was helping to facilitate local municipal health councils' required planning meetings and ensure that they were submitting their annual municipal health plan to the Ministry of Health. Each municipal health plan was supposed to include key information, such as what kind of health programing the municipal government was going to undertake the next year and its budget for each item. With Alicia, he was discussing the timeline for the meetings and the process for ensuring that municipalities would submit their plans.

Offhand moments like Ramón's phone call with Alicia highlighted for me the kinds of day-to-day coordinations required to put policy into practice. In this case, limited funding, personnel, and capacity for enforcement made it challenging for state officials to ensure that every single municipality in Bolivia would develop its own health plan. GHA had some funds to help convene the meetings required by national law in the municipalities where they worked. It was thus not unusual for NGOs like GHA to play a role in the implementation of state policy, even as MAS officials had declared that they wanted to move away from aid dependency and establish "national sovereignty" over health care (Johnson 2010).

As it sought to move away from neoliberal austerity measures, the Morales administration increased the revenues it could spend on social programs—including health care—by taxing oil and gas extraction in the lowlands. These measures were also controversial, as critics argued that the state's reliance on extractive development frequently eroded promised state protections for Indigenous sovereignty in the lowland regions of Bolivia.[18] But if numerous scholars and activists critiqued the decolonial state for its hypocrisy in eroding Indigenous rights, MAS officials often insisted that they were working with constrained choices and attempting to keep resource wealth in Bolivia for social services and infrastructures. Although the MAS largely maintained a capitalist system, it framed these investments as a turn away from prior neoliberal regimes, when foreign companies had funneled resource wealth out of Bolivia (Gustafson 2020). However, while overall health care spending increased under the Morales administration, it was not enough to counter resource shortages that were both longstanding and had been exacerbated through prior decades of privatization and state rollback of investment in social services—highlighting how an ostensibly postneoliberal era continued to be haunted by lingering neoliberal formations (Goodale and Postero 2013).[19]

In practice, the Morales administration, much like its predecessors, continued to rely on NGOs to help provide health care services—but it also sought to bring them more in line with a state agenda. Diana Cordoba and Kees Jansen (2016) note that as the Morales administration worked to reassert the role of the state in social service delivery, NGOs increasingly positioned themselves as being able to offer technical expertise and support for state projects. Thus, NGOs such as GHA, which worked in Machacamarca and surrounding areas, often coordinated closely with state officials to help implement national policies. The Bolivian branch of GHA was staffed entirely by Bolivians, several of whom had also previously worked for state and regional health institutions. In Machacamarca, GHA staffers regularly held workshops explaining the key tenets of the SAFCI policy to local biomedical practitioners. They provided logistical support for ministry-led workshops and local health planning events; they also helped collect documents (such as healers' patient records and household survey data) to facilitate state policy interventions. As in the case of the phone call with Ramón, they also helped ensure that municipal councils were meeting and developing annual health plans. In the day to day, the NGO functioned as an arm of the state, coordinating closely with state and regional health officials, even as it also brought its own funding priorities and framings.

Despite the fragmentary nature of the health care system and of policies themselves, warm care often emerged as a shared common ground, something that state officials and NGO workers alike could embrace as fundamentally good for patients. GHA, a large, globally renowned organization based in Europe, had a mandate to support access to health care for populations it described as vulnerable; its Bolivia branch focused specifically on improving care for women and Indigenous patients. Like many other international aid and human rights organizations, they took a more depoliticized approach to care that positioned universal rights and alleviation of suffering as central goals.[20] In contrast to the MAS's policy framing documents, NGO documents placed less discursive emphasis on social medicine, radical pluralism, or remaking conceptions of health itself. But GHA positioned their own focus on patient rights within a liberal paradigm as largely in alignment with the Morales administration's own projects of improving care, even if they rarely used terms such as "decolonization" in their own documents, workshops, and framings. These alignments highlighted not only how organizations like GHA sought to coordinate with the state, but also how ultimately the project of warm care had a broad appeal. Warm care, with its emphasis on cultural inclusion and humane treatment of patients, could easily be taken up as part of mainstream global health work.

Even so, several policymakers I interviewed worried that the Morales administration had stepped too far back from supporting the primary, preventative, and intercultural health care work central to the SAFCI and the Law of Traditional and Ancestral Medicine, as it left much of the on-the-ground work to NGOs. Instead, they noted, the MAS had increasingly turned its limited funds to investing in material infrastructures such as new second- and third-tier hospitals. In their view, new, modern hospital constructions looked good for the president in a context of historically underfunded infrastructure—but ultimately, such investments did little to care for the health of the majority of the population, who needed access to basic primary and preventative care. Such investments also did not address the broader problem of existing hospitals and health centers that were deeply underresourced.

Nonetheless, other state bureaucrats did see infrastructural investments—including new specialty hospital constructions, gifts of ambulances and medical equipment, and an extensive telehealth system that connected rural outposts to specialists in urban hospitals—as part of a decolonial project. State officials inaugurated new infrastructural projects in events replete with Indigenous social movement symbols—for example, by invoking the name and image of Aymara rebellion leader Túpac Katari for a new state satellite that would help support the telehealth network (Centellas, forthcoming). Describing how state officials invoked Indigenous social movement symbols in a gift of tractors for a rural community, Anders Burman (2017) notes that the Morales administration frequently reframed modernist development initiatives as part of an Indigenous decolonial project. Doing so signaled that the kinds of infrastructures that had long been denied Indigenous communities or used as an assimilationist tool of their improvement now belonged to them—were now being mobilized in their service (Centellas, forthcoming).

Divisions between these two perspectives (investments in infrastructure versus investments in primary care) were not always clear-cut. For example, state investments in the satellite-based telehealth network did in fact reach many smaller rural health posts and clinics, thereby expanding access to care for people who could not easily travel to more specialized hospitals in cities. I suggest that the Morales administration's shifts toward investing in and publicizing infrastructures were also simultaneously a means to signal to a wider public that officials were using resources to the good; that is, they were caring for the population in a way that prior regimes of neoliberal austerity had not. State performances and opening ceremonies were central, not only to reminding the public of the state's decolonial commitments (Postero 2017), but also to affirming the narrative of a caring state.

These circulations pointed to how warm care could be invoked in different ways at different moments. In one instance, the highly publicized construction of urban specialty hospitals could be framed as signs of a caring state. In another, NGO workshops emphasizing individual and group-based rights could also be framed as continuous with this same state project of care. While policy implementation was often diffuse and fragmentary, institutional actors continually worked to emphasize that the Morales administration offered a new era of care by including, rendering visible, and centering Indigenous patient experiences in public institutions. Warm care could be invoked in different (if overlapping) ways by different institutional actors, and yet it worked to create points of alignment that largely sustained the existing working of institutions.

As David Mosse points out, even if policy is frequently incoherent, part of the work of bureaucrats is to make it retroactively appear coherent; projects "work to maintain themselves as coherent policy ideas, as systems of representations as well as operational systems" (2004, 654–55).[21] To return to the scene that opened this chapter: when questioned about the disjuncture between policy rhetoric and implementation during the traditional medicine roundtable I attended, Alonzo continually sought to bring the narrative back to the state's decolonial project. Even as participants questioned and criticized the implementation of intercultural health policies, he narrated these critiques as part of the state's decolonial process; he reminded participants that the very act of doing a roundtable was a way to ensure that they were elaborating programs that centered their demands. In a context of constrained resources and patchy implementation, warm care also became a way for state officials and institutions to signal that they still cared—that they were working to include Indigenous voices and perspectives in the state. Warmth was central to reaffirming the narrative of an attentive and inclusive state under Evo Morales, even when resources were scarce, even when access to care remained uneven.

As I will show throughout this book, this extension of state care could be a meaningful point of engagement, which Indigenous patients, healers, and community members could also rework toward their own ends. However, it did not necessarily break from the ways that bureaucratic state systems enacted structural violence and intensified the regulation of Indigenous bodies, relations, and practices. Instead, I suggest that warm care enabled new kinds of obfuscations. In folding back into existing ways of doing health—which heavily sought to fix, regulate, and intervene in Indigenous life—health reforms largely sidestepped addressing the historical and structural drivers of illness, including land dispossession, material inequality, and racism. Instead, in affirming a narrative of a newly caring, inclusive state, it positioned the state itself as innocent in ongoing colonial processes (see also Rivera Cusicanqui 2014; Winchell 2022).

In 2013, I attended an event sponsored by the WHO and the PAHO in the city center of La Paz titled "Workshop Seminar Encounter Between Biomedicine and Traditional Medicine." Entering the dimly lit auditorium, I took my seat in the crowded rows of chairs alongside healers, biomedical practitioners, NGO workers, and state officials. A poster, placed on the front stage, showed a biomedical doctor and a traditional healer facing the camera and shaking hands. To open the event, Alberto Camaqui, the Vice-Minister of Traditional Medicine and Interculturality, came up to the stage to give a speech. As he faced his audience, he pronounced starkly, "We still live in a colonized state, with colonized ministries. We are still oppressed. We do not have the same rights or support as other ministries. Decolonization, for the moment, has not advanced [la descolonización por el momento se quedó ahí]."

I would be reminded of the speech when, nearly a year later, Camaqui emphasized at the roundtable held at the AECID offices that transnational NGOs had been the only ones to support traditional healers. As I learned from interviewing him, Camaqui was a proponent of enacting state-led decolonization in health care—but he worried that not enough resources had been allocated to making the project a reality. The vice-minister's narrative about the endurance of colonialism presented a stark contrast to the hopeful outline Alonzo proposed. For Alonzo, the state was in the process of rupturing with a colonial past; for the vice-minister, colonialism endured despite promises of transformation and was reproduced within the state apparatus itself.

Throughout this chapter, I have examined how MAS policymakers framed the project of decolonizing health care as one that might offer a "new way of thinking, feeling, and doing health" that could rupture with past colonial and neoliberal capitalist modes of intervention. On paper, policymakers emphasized the centrality of radical pluralism, sustaining relational well-being (Vivir Bien), and reimagining services to center Indigenous epistemologies, ontologies, and ethics. Yet, as I have shown, resource constraints and the routing of policy transformation through existing institutions often meant that policy implementation took a different form than what was written on paper—leading to critiques like the one developed by the vice-minister. Moving away from the idea of decolonization as radical undoing, policymakers, NGO workers, and others involved with policy reform increasingly came to emphasize Indigenous ontologies and epistemologies in terms of their warm, caring aspects. This shift allowed state officials to promise care and inclusion for Bolivia's previously excluded, majority Indigenous and poor population—but did not necessarily entail major transformation of the basic premises of biomedicine and public health. In the following chapters, I trace how these reinscriptions played out on the ground in Machacamarca, with varying effects for health, the body, and care in practice.

2 REORIENTING CARE

Benevolence, Violence, and Medical Training

"I always asked myself where the word 'patient' comes from. Now I understand, patient comes from treating with patience. You have to treat patients with patience. So that the patient trusts you. So that the patient feels protected. When the doctor treats you with cariño [affection, care], you can almost heal yourself with his words. You already feel sure that you will be cured."
— PRESIDENT EVO MORALES AYMA, quoted on the cover page
for the SAFCI course textbook
(Ministerio de Salud de Bolivia 2014, 5, my translation)

ONE AFTERNOON, IN THE MAIN meeting room of the Machacamarca Hospital, Dr. Lydia asked the hospital staff to perform skits about how health care had changed since Evo Morales was elected president of Bolivia. A doctor working for the Ministry of Health, she traveled once a week over several months to Machacamarca to teach hospital workers about the SAFCI policy. Most days, the doctors and nurses participating in the course gave PowerPoint presentations of chapters from the textbook, reciting what they had read in a monotone to a dozing audience. Today, Dr. Lydia decided to change things up. She had the hospital workers divide into groups and perform a short play about what they had learned.

The first to perform was a group of five doctors—close friends who always sat in the back of class and whispered to one another. They cleared the front of the room save a small table, and Dr. César, an obstetrics and gynecology resident, donned his white coat. On a blank piece of paper, he scribbled the words "Dr. $US" and taped it to his chest. He then swaggered over—his stride long and exaggerated—to the small table, taking a seat next to Dr. Estela, who was playing the nurse. She twirled her hair slowly around her finger and stared at her phone.

Dr. Reinaldo and Dr. Fany stumbled onto the improvised stage, wearing their own paper labels that read *pobre*, or "poor person." Dr. Reinaldo cried out that his "sister" had terrible stomach pains. On cue, Dr. Fany moaned loudly and clutched her stomach.

"Do you have money to pay?" demanded "Dr. $US."

"We'll find the money," Reinaldo replied, agitated. "Please help my sister!"

"Fine. Go check her vitals," "Dr. $US" instructed the "nurse." She rolled her eyes and reluctantly tore herself from her phone. She strode over to where Fany was sitting, still clutching her stomach. She roughly prodded her "patient," eliciting cries of pain. Rolling her eyes again, the "nurse" announced that everything seemed fine.

"Dr. $US" turned toward his "patient." "You probably have appendicitis and will need an operation," he told her imperiously. "It will cost you a lot of money."

The door to the auditorium opened again, and Dr. Mayra rushed in wearing a label that read *rica*, or "rich person." "I hurt my nail!" she wailed. "Dr. $US" and the "nurse" immediately rushed to her side, arms flailing, crying out that this was an emergency. They promised her all the best care and medications they had at their disposal.

At this point, the doctors paused their skit. Their over-the-top, comedic delivery had the audience bent over laughing. Dr. César, who played the villainous "Dr. $US," began explaining more seriously that this was how the capitalist system worked. Patients were treated as clients, and money would buy you better care. He announced that now, the group would perform the health care system the government was trying to create. They switched out their paper labels for new ones that all read *iguales*, or "equals." They acted out the same scenario as before, but this time, when the poor siblings entered the room, the doctor and nurse greeted them with a friendly, "Buen día." The doctor kindly asked them what the matter was, and the nurse gently measured the patient's blood pressure. Afterwards, the doctor wrote a prescription and explained to the patient that she could get her medications for free at the pharmacy. When the formerly "rich" patient came in, they politely told her she would have to wait her turn.

This chapter traces what policymakers described as efforts to "reorient" health services (*reorientar los servicios de salud*), largely by encouraging practitioners to adopt moral practices of attentiveness and treating all patients equally. Training courses, like the one run by Dr. Lydia in the Machacamarca Hospital, were designed to transform modes of care from a system of discrimination to one of equality, from inaccessibility to accessibility, from harshness and mistreatment to *cariño*. Such training programs were also diffuse, offered infrequently and in a piecemeal fashion as workshops or continuing education courses. At the time of my research, they were rarely integrated into university medical training, which, with a few exceptions, continued to focus primarily on the biological and clinical, rather than the social, dimensions of medicine.

In Machacamarca, Dr. Lydia's SAFCI training course became a site where, on occasion, practitioners might articulate aspirations, might narrate and imagine ideal forms of equitable care. Both Dr. César and Dr. Reinaldo had studied at the Latin American School of Medicine (*Escuela Latinoamericana de Medicina*, ELAM) in Havana, Cuba, before returning to Bolivia to complete their required rural residency; they were two out of three doctors employed at the Machacamarca Hospital who had done so. In the context of the ministry training course, they quickly grasped the textbook sections on the social determinants of health, frequently referring back to their own prior training in Cuba to supplement discussion. Yet they were not the only ones who latched onto this discussion. Many Bolivia-trained practitioners working in the Machacamarca Hospital were newer to these concepts, yet they similarly pointed to the problems of unequal access to care. The character of "Dr. $US" satirized the exclusions of capitalist health care and articulated an anti-imperialist critique of the U.S. government's global export of privatized models of health care, particularly through its aid programs and its support for structural adjustment measures. For many biomedical practitioners in the Machacamarca Hospital, the desired imaginary of good care involved accessibility and equal treatment, regardless of social class.

Even so, day-to-day practices of care in the hospital often looked very different from the imaginary of good care articulated in the skit. While it did not necessarily replicate the cartoonish representation of exclusionary care from the first half of the skit, hospital-based care often continued to reinscribe profound raced, classed, and gendered hierarchies. Underpaid and precariously employed practitioners often continued to shift the problems of material shortages onto patient bodies themselves as they expressed concerns about patient ignorance and noncompliance. Moves toward warm care—such as showing kindness, treating patients equally, and being attentive to patients' circumstances—folded back into long-standing linkages between benevolence and violence in the clinic. Residents of Machacamarca frequently described their local hospital as a place *donde no hay atención* ("where there is no treatment" or "where there is no care")—a phrase that encapsulated both material dearth and problems of mistreatment and neglect. For many patients, conditions of "no care" were experienced in a range of ways—sometimes, as verging on the murderous (Stevenson 2014), other times as inspiring minor affects of anxiety, irritation, and ambivalence (Ngai 2005) that led to a slow wearing down.

What to make, then, of a seeming division between ideals and practice in biomedical caregiving in the Machacamarca Hospital? How did care that practitioners aspired to make inclusive end up being exclusionary for patients? In Chapter 1, I examined critiques—coming especially from traditional healers—about divisions between "just talk" and "actually doing something" with policy. I traced how activist state bureaucrats confronted the limitations of change as they navigated the intersections of material scarcity and entrenched colonial, capitalist, and liberal structures. In this chapter, I extend these points to argue that a similar dynamic of navigating constrained resources and working with existing categories unfolded within the space of the hospital itself, reproduced especially through habituated clinical care practice. In other words, routinized practices of care in a context of resource shortages had long sustained hierarchies in the clinic. And while the training course and the skit offered opportunities for imagining a world otherwise, they were also not set up to tackle the conditions that reinforced inequality in practice. Instead, I suggest, discourses of warm care and inclusion could often—and seemingly paradoxically— deflect from the very conditions that constrained care in the clinic.

Attention to routinized, embodied care practice shifts the focus away from individual intentions and toward broader structures that naturalized racist and racializing projects in the clinic. I argue that everyday practices of providing for others in the clinic remained tied to colonial modes of benevolence that situated providers and patients in different ways within linked racial and class hierarchies. For precariously situated biomedical practitioners, practicing medical authority in the clinic solidified class mobility and proximity to whiteness. In turn, patients, by virtue of seeking out care at a rural public institution, were racialized as more Indigenous—and therefore, in need of charity, intervention, and regulation. The idea that unruly patients needed to be urged to collaborate in biomedical regimes was deeply ingrained in practitioners' care practices.

Care in the clinic was also inextricable from a context of material inequality and constrained resources. As practitioners themselves struggled with precarious employment and medical equipment shortages, they often felt powerless to push back against the structures that put them in a difficult position. Instead, falling back onto habituated action also became a way to shift blame for medicine not working onto patients. I dwell on how entrenched structural violence in medicine can also generate forms of obfuscation that ultimately hide the conditions contributing to inequality and shift blame onto those with less power.

By foregrounding routinized care practice in the clinic, I work to understand how habits can persist despite rhetoric otherwise. The SAFCI training course, I suggest, became a key site where tensions (and obfuscations) around structural change emerged. On the one hand, the course encouraged biomedical practitioners to reflect on key structural questions of patient access and the effects of neoliberal privatization on health services. Yet opportunities like the skit also became a site for practitioners to act out an idealized form of warm care where resource shortages were seemingly not a factor and patients fully desired practitioners' interventions. While a central ground of ethical aspiration for practitioners, the skit also sidestepped questions of how race and class inequality—produced through layered projects of colonialism and capitalism—continued to matter for everyday clinical practice.

This chapter thus examines how moves toward warm care in the clinic extended and sometimes reinvented long-standing racialized presuppositions in new forms—reflecting how, as Carmen Alvaro Jarrín puts it, "biopolitical discourses about race have an uncanny way of refashioning themselves into new shapes" (2017, 13). I begin this chapter with a discussion of how race and class hierarchies were produced in clinical practice. I then shift to a discussion of how efforts to reorient care were refracted across multiple sites. Toggling ethnographically between training programs and clinical practice points to the piecemeal nature of (re)training, how new orientations can coexist with old, and how training programs may themselves include framings that reinscribe the various processes they seek to undo. Amid these configurations, warm care became tied to doing good and treating all patients equally, but also reinscribed the idea that Aymara patients were noncompliant and needed to be disciplined into the space of the clinic.

BECOMING A BIOMEDICAL PRACTITIONER

In keeping with the town of Machacamarca's status as a small regional hub, the municipal hospital was constructed in 2001 to serve residents of the town and surrounding villages, replacing a smaller health center. It was staffed mainly by general medical practitioners and nurses who provided primary care and emergency services. In addition, a small rotating group of medical residents—doing their year of obligatory rural service as part of their residency programs—offered more specialized services such as pediatrics, gynecology, internal medicine, and minor surgeries. Finally, the hospital also employed several key support staff, including a social worker, a lab technician, an X-ray technician, a statistician, an administrator, two cooks, two janitors, and a groundskeeper. The wider municipality of Machaca-marca also had three primary care health posts, located in smaller rural villages some distance from the main town. Each health post was staffed by a nurse or a general medical practitioner.

In Bolivia, working as a biomedical provider—especially in public clinics and hospitals—could be a precarious profession. Specialist doc-tors (such as gynecologists, surgeons) usually found work in the cities, and they sometimes held down two jobs—one at a large public hospital and one at a (better paying) private clinic—to make ends meet. Gen-eral medical practitioners and nurses, however, were usually funneled into primary care clinics and small hospitals like the one in Machaca-marca. They were often from slightly lower income backgrounds than their specialist colleagues. A number of those who worked in Macha-camarca were also descended from Aymara migrants to the city of El Alto. General practitioners also had more difficulty finding work, in part because there were more medical and nursing students graduat-ing than positions available.

One morning, I was sitting in the hospital's general consultation room with Dr. Mayra, who had played the role of the rich patient in the skit. It was nearing noon, and the influx of patients had slowed. Nieves, the nurse, had momentarily stepped out, and Dr. Mayra and I made small talk—she, sitting behind the creaky metal desk and I, perched on a high, spindly stool in the corner. I asked her how long she had been working in the hospital.

"Nine months," she replied. "I was happy to get this job." She began to recount her difficulties finding work. When she graduated medical school, she had been unable to find a paid position, so she took an unpaid one at a rural clinic to build up her resume. She could not sur-vive long without a salary, however, so she soon took a job at a phar-macy in the city of Oruro. Yet she still wanted to work as a doctor, so after a year, she responded to a job posting in the municipality of Machacamarca. The position was for a doctor for one of the municipal health posts, located in a village several kilometers from the town of Machacamarca. But when she arrived, municipal government officials informed her they could not employ her because another doctor, one trained in Cuba, had already come to work there. (As I later learned, the doctor was employed through the state-funded Mi Salud program, meaning that the municipal government did not have to pay for the post). Dr. Mayra went to complain to the mayor, and fortunately, he offered her a position at the Machacamarca Hospital.

Dr. Mayra had finally found stable employment, but her pay continued to arrive irregularly. Some time after our conversation, I found her and Dr. Estela complaining that they had not received a paycheck in months, because the municipal government's accounts were frozen. During the transition to a new mayor, the central government put local funds on hold to prevent the outgoing mayor's staff from taking any money. This hold, however, lasted several months. It disrupted the pay of hospital workers (including doctors, nurses, administrators, and cleaning and maintenance staff) and the daily functioning of the hospital (for example, the ambulance could not run because there was no money for gasoline). Such incidents made it so that hospital workers received their salaries in fits and starts, making for precarious living.

For most of the practitioners I came to know, a position in Machacamarca was a temporary step toward a better one. They commuted to the small town several times a week on the rickety mini-bus from El Alto, sleeping in the chilly dorms behind the hospital only when they worked double shifts. When I returned for a follow-up visit six months after completing my research, many of the doctors and nurses I had known there were gone. When I returned a year after that, all of them were gone, replaced by an entirely new staff. Most had found positions closer to home in El Alto and La Paz.

Yet despite the precariousness of their working conditions, nurses and doctors often marked themselves as being from a different social class than their patients, even when they shared rural Aymara roots. Being a *profesional* (a university educated, salaried worker) and having

access to biomedical expertise often allowed them to position themselves as mestizo or simply unmarked, rather than Indigenous.[1] As
scholars have noted, race in the Andes is often malleable, constituted
through social and material markers such as class, education, language, and dress, even as racial discrimination based on phenotype
also endures.[2] Amid the legacies of national projects of mestizaje, factors such as speaking Spanish, access to education, and living in a city
can also grant one proximity to whiteness.

For many practitioners, efforts to be socially mobile took shape
against the backdrop of rural-to-urban migration in Bolivia. Many
Aymara migrants to El Alto and La Paz one or two generations ago
worried about facing discrimination and encouraged their children to
assimilate, especially when it came to language. Most of my interlocutors who were medical practitioners never learned to speak Aymara,
even when their parents or grandparents spoke the language. During
a later interview with Dr. Mayra, she described how her parents spoke
Aymara, but insisted that she learn English as her second language
alongside Spanish. Similarly, a friend of mine in La Paz lamented she
had not taught her daughter Aymara, because now her daughter had
to take Aymara language classes to become a nurse.

Becoming a medical professional was a means of obtaining social
mobility through dominant ways of knowing. Yet efforts to solidify
racial and class positions also unfolded through the hierarchies of
labor in the hospital. Doctors, nurses, and various support staff (social
workers, laboratory technicians, administrators) inhabited different
social positions in the hospital, even as they shared concerns about
the precarity of their professions and their ability to practice medicine
effectively. General medicine doctors were in a position of authority
to make decisions, and despite the irregularities of their income, they
were also slightly better paid. Nurses and support staff, including
social workers and laboratory technicians, were paid less. Nurses, especially, were more likely to speak Aymara, and they often took on an
intermediary role. During clinical visits, they both aided with medical tasks (measuring and weighing patients, retrieving instruments,

injecting flu shots) and translated between doctors and monolingual Aymara patients.

COLLABORATION AND NONCOLLABORATION

It was not the first or last time I would hear a doctor tell a patient, "¡No me estás colaborando!" (idiomatic Bolivian Spanish for "You are not collaborating!" or "You are not helping me!"). Dr. César was attending to an Aymara woman in labor who was crying out from severe pain, and who (seemingly) was not pushing as he had instructed her to push. If she did not "collaborate"—if she did not do her part—the baby would not come out, he warned her.

Dr. César was a charismatic doctor who had come up with much of the script he and his fellow doctors performed for the training course. He also came from a low-income Aymara family from the city of El Alto. Informed in part by his prior training at the ELAM in Cuba, he was a great believer in equality of access and the kinds of community-based, primary care work the SAFCI proposed to enact. Yet he worried that, even as it was written in the law, there were few opportunities to do the preventative and educational work he saw as central to improving health. As a gynecologist, he worried women were not receiving good guidance about pregnancy and childbirth and that he was seeing them for the first time when they came into labor at the hospital. As he put it, patients still clung to nonscientific beliefs. "Unfortunately, the idiosyncrasy of our population also says a lot," he told me. "We have lived five hundred years oppressed under colonialism and we still continue to be oppressed. We maintain this way of thinking, or this idiosyncrasy—that doctors are not good, that *naturistas* and *Kallawayas* and *curanderos* [different kinds of traditional healer] are better."

Although he also situated himself in the "we" of living five hundred years oppressed under colonialism, he framed the impacts of colonialism differently than the structural and historical critique of power proposed by many activists and state officials. In Dr. César's narration, colonial oppression was the root cause of "idiosyncratic" ways of thinking and lack of trust in biomedical doctors. His words pointed in part to the heterogeneity of perspectives on indigeneity and colonialism in Bolivia; there was not always a neat consensus. But they also echoed a broader pattern (across many practitioners I interviewed) of emphasizing patients' ignorance and noncompliance as central barriers to care. If many practitioners took workshop messaging to heart and emphasized their commitment to equality of access, they often described their frustration that patients seemingly did not desire the care that they were providing.

The phrase "No me estás colaborando" would come to haunt my field research—as would another one: *Es por tu bien* ("It is for your own good"). From many providers' perspectives, such chastisements were a key component of good care provision, particularly in a context of diagnostic and material uncertainty. Clinicians I interviewed worried about the precarious conditions of their own labor, as well as the limited supply of medications and equipment that made both diagnosis and treatment more difficult. Like many public institutions, the Machacamarca Hospital had long been underfunded—a condition produced through layered histories of both national and global divestment from health care, exacerbated through structural adjustment policies and their aftereffects (see Chapter 1). In addition, given the Machacamarca Hospital's status as a small hospital mostly focused on primary care and emergency services, providers worried that they could not treat more complex problems in the hospital itself. Instead, they worked to stabilize patients with more intricate conditions and transfer them to larger hospitals in the cities of La Paz or El Alto.

As in many contexts with constrained resources (Livingston 2012; Street 2014), biomedical providers worked to improvise solutions and develop situated forms of judgment and expertise to treat patients. Providers often found alternative workarounds when the technologies they needed were not available—for example, by substituting equipment or building their own sling to hold a broken arm until a patient could obtain a full cast in La Paz. As Alice Street (2014) has powerfully demonstrated, in contexts of constrained resources, diagnostic closure is not always possible—and clinicians may see the patient body itself as partially unknowable, as obstructive to the biomedical gaze. For providers in the Machacamarca hospital, constrained resources were both a pragmatic reality underpinning their care work and a source of frequent commentary and frustration. In chastising patients, providers sought to encourage patients to participate correctly in the medical encounter—thereby making tenuous connections come together more smoothly and facilitating the process of diagnosis and treatment.

Scholarship on the prevalence of medical paternalism in Latin America has likewise demonstrated how clinicians frequently understand chastisement to be a form of care—one that helps foster responsibility in patients and thereby also facilitates their healing.[3] In some contexts, patients themselves may also accept chastisement or see it as a caring practice—for example, because it helps create certainty in a context of uncertainty (Singer 2022). For many patients I interviewed in Machacamarca, medical paternalism was an expected, even appropriate, practice of care—a sign of providers' attention and far preferable to experiences of neglect patients also frequently experienced in public institutions (see also Roberts 2012). But chastisement itself was the subject of more ambivalence—and sometimes outright criticism. In Chapter 5, I return to this question by tracing how many patients did not seek individual autonomy in the medical encounter or to fully disrupt medical authority, but they did hope that providers might use their position of authority in ways that demonstrated personalized attention and long-term, often material, commitments to patients and their families. To this end, many patients praised providers who they saw as *cariñoso* (caring, affectionate)—a suggestion also raised in the president's quote that opened this chapter, but that many patients saw not just as a momentary act of kindness, but a practice of extended labor and attention. In contrast, when providers berated patients, patients often sat in silence in the moment, not responding to the provider's words. Yet afterwards, they complained to family members and friends about their provider's treatment of them—a dynamic I came to understand better as I also spent more time outside of the hospital. For instance, one of my neighbors, Evangelina, complained at length about her experiences with a hospital social worker who had berated her and accused her of lying about the circumstances of her grandson, who was a patient in the hospital. For her and others, practitioners' harsh treatment often contributed to what they described as an experience of "no care" in the hospital.

Attending to these practices, I suggest, highlights how structural violence can be enacted through habituated action—when, as Felicity Aulino suggests, the very systems that revolve around providing for others are ones that "maintain inequity and oppression" (2019, 142). I argue that providers' concerns about material uncertainty and encouraging patients to participate correctly in the medical encounter were also inseparable from the racialization of Indigenous patient bodies as inherently unruly. Put differently, the question of whose body might be deemed especially obstructive to the biomedical gaze was inseparable from the histories and structures that had long positioned biomedicine as a site of modernization and racial assimilation. As Khiara Bridges notes, clinical encounters are key sites for ongoing dialectical processes of race and class formation. In her study of a New York hospital, she highlights how medical practices and systems constitute low-income, racially minoritized women as having "unruly bodies" and posing "threats to the body politic" (2011, 16) (see also Davis 2019). Resonantly, in numerous Latin American contexts, scholars have shown how, even as biomedicine has been held up as a tool of social whitening under regimes of mestizaje, low-income patients in public clinics are often perceived by practitioners as "more Indigenous" and therefore also more unruly.[4] As Margarita Huayhua points out, in neighboring Peru, clinical encounters are especially prime sites for linguistic racism—where through communicative care practices, rural Indigenous patients are often construed as more animal-like, "put[ting] in question their status as human beings capable of decisions about their health, well-being, and any other aspect that concerns them" (2013, 53). While providers frequently expressed concerns that patients in the Machacamarca area were noncompliant, they especially directed these concerns toward patients who they read as more Indigenous, including patients who were monolingual Aymara speakers, low income, or from more rural surrounding villages in the municipality. Practi-

tioners especially scolded patients they perceived as not listening to
their instructions, or who they suspected would not come back for all
of their required follow-up visits.

Understanding such practices as intimately bound up in habituated norms of care in the clinic also highlights how providers themselves were brought into race-making projects. As I noted previously,
biomedical providers came from a range of backgrounds—including
some (like Dr. César and Dr. Mayra) whose parents spoke Aymara. If
being a biomedical practitioner in general could position one as an
upwardly mobile subject, the repetition of verbal and embodied practices of chastisement also became a way to absorb practitioners into
unmarked whiteness.[5] I suggest that in this context, the social workings of race were both obfuscated and obfuscating. As Aymara political
theorist Carlos Macusaya Cruz (2020) has noted, in Bolivia race often
goes unnamed and the very existence of racism denied—a legacy of
the myth of mestizaje that simultaneously positions everyone as "just
Bolivians" while continuing to code difference through phenotype,
language, dress, geography, gender, income, and more (see also de
la Cadena 2000; Molina 2021). Such obfuscations, I suggest, allowed
routine clinical practices to be naturalized as good care, as preoccupation with patient well-being that might make biomedicine work more
effectively. Simultaneously, focusing on the racialized noncompliance
of patient bodies also obfuscated the material conditions of the clinic
that made care difficult. While economically precarious providers
acknowledged problems of underfunding, it was often easier to shift
blame for biomedicine not working onto patients themselves rather
than onto the seemingly immovable social and material structures of
the clinic. Habituated care practice sustained orderings that largely localized barriers to treatment within patient bodies and comportments.

WORK AND PLAY

Dr. Lydia traveled from La Paz to the Machacamarca Hospital to offer
a biweekly training course over a period of several months. She had
received the position with the ministry as the doctor in charge of the

SAFCI for the health district because she herself had undertaken a SAFCI residency—a new residency established under the new law, specifically teaching doctors to focus on community health. But in her current position, her role was mostly that of administrator. She collected paperwork and traveled sporadically to Machacamarca to give the course that would bring hospital practitioners up to speed on the new policies, based on a formal textbook and program set out by the ministry.

Efforts to transform the conditions of clinical care have been a key component of leftist social medicine projects in Latin America, as policy reformers worked to link the health of the body to the health of the nation (Brotherton 2012; Cooper 2019). In the wake of the Pink Tide that swept across Latin America in the early 2000s, especially, elements of Cuban medical training fanned outwards to other countries. Cuban medical practitioners provided humanitarian aid, students from other countries went to study at the ELAM, and the country's models of health care were adopted more widely.⁶ In these contexts, reformers positioned practitioner-patient interactions as microcosms of wider goals of justice and egalitarianism. Alissa Bernstein (2013) considers how Bolivian doctors studying at the ELAM in Cuba were trained to adopt socially and politically oriented clinical subjectivities in their medical practice that they then brought back to Bolivia with them—echoes of which also reverberated through Dr. César and Dr. Reinaldo's narratives. Amy Cooper (2019) resonantly describes how, in the context of the Barrio Adentro health program during Hugo Chávez's presidency in Venezuela, practitioners (many of whom had come from Cuba) were expected to show kindness and compassion to patients—a significant shift from prior forms of mistreatment in public clinics. As Cooper demonstrates, this set of expectations around biomedical care diverges from modes of medical training in the United States—where, as medical anthropologists have shown, competence is often seen as being in tension with care (Good and Good 1993) and the biomedical practitioner is assumed to be a "divided self" (Kleinman 2011). Rather, in these regionally circulating models for transforming care, attentiveness is intimately tied to both biomedical treatment and treating the social body as a whole.

It was a mode of orienting care that also came to inform home-grown Bolivian efforts to retrain medical practitioners—but also with some key differences. In contrast to Cuba and Venezuela, Bolivian health reforms were less sweeping, and efforts to transform providers' approaches were more diffuse and fragmentary. For example, certification courses like the one that Dr. Lydia ran were offered sporadically and were not integrated into medical training from the start. The patchwork implementation reflected prior decades of underfunding, embedded within global resource flows as well as projects of structural adjustment; it also reflected the Morales administration's prioritization of how to use limited funds (see Chapter 1).

Another key difference was that other leftist state moves to recraft care largely focused on class as the basis for inclusion in health care systems—where, for example, kind and compassionate care in Venezuelan low-income neighborhoods was linked to broader populist reforms (Cooper 2019). In contrast, in Bolivia, training programs, much like wider policies, directly linked Indigenous struggle with class struggle, anticolonialism with anticapitalism. Therefore, the course textbook also asked biomedical practitioners to think through how to provide care that was inclusive on multiple fronts—that was accessible, egalitarian, and attentive to cultural differences. Yet, much like health policy itself, this intersectional framing took on a much more limited form in the context of training programs. As I will show, efforts to teach this framing to practitioners were abstracted from day-to-day medical practice and sidestepped confrontations with enduring dynamics of race and constrained resources in the health care setting.

As part of the official Ministry of Health course run by Dr. Lydia, participants were offered grades and a certification at the end. The class was packed full—for, in a context of uncertain employment, medical practitioners frequently sought programs with certifications to build up their resumes. The course offered a broad overview of medical practice in the context of the SAFCI policy. Beyond explanations of specific reforms, the core ministry textbook drew connections to national and global economic processes, political philosophies, and social movements. Dr. Lydia structured the course around the textbook, so that each class session covered a different chapter. These had such titles as "Healthcare as a Political Process," "Decolonization and Living Well," and "The Global Crisis of Capitalism." Like national policy itself, the content of the text blended multiple approaches and styles. Theories from Marx, Hegel, and Bourdieu were woven into the text to describe the workings of power and inequality. Interspersed between the chapters were paintings of key Indigenous resistance leaders since Spanish colonization (for example, Túpac Katari, Bartolina Sisa) with short biographies underneath.

Other portions of the textbook, in turn, emphasized the importance of kindness and warmth toward patients—namely, the need to center *calidad y calidez* (quality and warmth) and *cariño*—a term that loosely translates to "affection" or "care." In the epigraph that opens this chapter, President Morales is directly quoted in the training textbook articulating the importance of cariño. I am less concerned with the etymology of the word "patient" than with what his interpretation implies: that practicing with patience, affection, and warmth can make patients feel supported and protected; it can even help patients start to heal. Quality and warmth in the clinic were closely tied to a broader project of political transformation.

Yet despite the activist framing of many of the assigned readings, the tenor of the class itself was often monotonous. Dr. Lydia rarely lectured, but during each session, she asked a small group of participants to prepare a PowerPoint summarizing the day's readings for the rest of the class. I sat in the back of the cramped meeting room, taking notes and watching groups of doctors and nurses present on their assigned chapters. They repeated what they had read almost verbatim and copied large blocks of text, charts, and definitions onto the slides. The other participants in the course drooped their eyes or, occasionally, got up to check on a patient across the hall. Observing that I was vigilantly taking notes on the course content, fellow coursetakers often asked to copy my answers on homework assignments and quizzes. When Dr. Lydia was not present, many participants grumbled that the course was too abstract—that it was "nice to learn about history," but what relevance did it have for the daily realities of medical practice in the hospital?

Such scenes of boredom might not be entirely unfamiliar to anyone who teaches for a living. Yet such responses were not inherently a reflection of disinterest or resistance. Writing in the context of Soviet Russia, for example, Alexei Yurchak (2013) describes how people sometimes fell asleep during Soviet Committee meetings—but nonetheless also remained hopeful about the promise of socialism itself. Participants in the course who I interviewed did not go so far as fully embracing the state project of reform—but they latched on to those elements of the course that aligned with the transformations that they themselves wanted to see in care.

During interviews, many biomedical practitioners described themselves as pro SAFCI—regardless of whether they were pro Evo Morales. Specifically, they supported the expansion of primary and preventative care, as well as increased access to services for patients. While this perspective was not necessarily shared by all doctors in Bolivia—the College of Physicians, as I noted in Chapter 1, initially opposed the SAFCI (Johnson 2010)—for at least a good number of practitioners in Machacamarca, experienced in working in a rural hospital, the SAFCI became also a means to extend the reach of biomedicine. Although many questioned the policy's focus on interculturality (see Chapter 3), they emphasized the importance of making biomedicine available for all.

If class readings, according to students, were largely "boring" and "irrelevant," the skit was a place to imagine a world in which such care was possible. The prompt for the skit was relatively open-ended: describe the differences between the past health care system and the health care system we are currently building. Most practitioners in the room presented a similar skit; they highlighted prior forms of mistreatment and contrasted these with present changes. Yet the skit was also an idealized moment of moral experimentation, deracinated from social and material context—wherein resource shortages in the clinic were seemingly not a factor and all patients appeared to ardently desire biomedical care. Warmth and attentiveness were also central to the provision of good care in this aspirational vision. As numerous practitioners emphasized to me—in interviews, off-hand conversations, and meetings—it was important to treat every patient who came in "with quality and warmth."

Anthropologists who study care and moral practice more broadly have often debated the relationship between ethics as tacit practice versus ethics as a site of abstracted discussion. Some have distinguished the everyday, habitual, and tacit workings of moral practice and the more explicitly articulated, reflective ethics of what one should do or how one should be (Robbins 2009; Lambek 2010). Others, however, have highlighted continuums between these different registers, as moments of reflection, abstraction, or speaking about what one should be doing may invite reconsideration of a practice or shift modes of attention (Brodwin 2013; Black 2018). Krista Van Vleet, for example, argues that interactive workshops and courses for single mothers at an NGO in Peru are key sites of moral apprenticeship; in social spaces like the workshop, "[y]oung women explore, normalize, and transform ethical and affective engagements and subjectivities" (2019, 60).

My conversations with biomedical practitioners in the Machacamarca hospital highlighted how they likewise used the space to engage in self-reflection and experiment with ethical possibilities. And yet, they also struggled to mobilize what they learned there in day-to-day clinical practice. As I show in the following, one lesson that practitioners embraced from the course was the need to be warmer and kinder to patients and to treat all patients equally. But practitioners still struggled with limited resources and continued to express concerns about patient noncompliance, funneling warm care through existing practices and assumptions about how to intervene in patient bodies. Notably, the training course did not ask practitioners to confront the kinds of choices they had to make when their resources were constrained—for example, when the very capitalist systems the textbook named had long choked state funding for clinics. It also did not ask them to confront the workings of racial hierarchies and their own place within them. Instead, the idealized imagery of the skit and the textbook allowed practitioners to imagine a world in which problems were already fixed.

WARM CARE AS REINSCRIPTION

One morning, I sat in the hospital's general consultation room with Dr. Mayra as she saw to her patients. Sitting behind the worn metal desk, she gestured to her patient, a hunched, elderly man named Leonardo, to take a seat across from her. "Kunas ustamxa?" she asked in slightly botched Aymara, recalling a phrase she had learned in her state-mandated language class. "What ails you?"

Leonardo placed his hands on his stomach and explained, in wavering Spanish, that his stomach hurt when he ate. The doctor nodded and politely instructed him (also in Spanish) to lie down on the exam table in the corner. He hobbled over to the table and clumsily climbed up. He stretched out with his hands behind the nape of his neck, as if relaxing on a bed.

Dr. Mayra shook her head. "No, no, put your hands down by your side." Leonardo moved his hands hesitantly. Dr. Mayra motioned again with her own hands stretched down, and he followed suit.

The doctor pressed down gently but firmly several times on Leonardo's abdomen, asking him if it hurt when she did so. He winced and nodded. After repeating the pressing motion several times, she told him to follow her back to the desk. She took a seat and scribbled a prescription for omeprazole, telling him to take one a day with breakfast and avoid heavy foods. She did not tell him his diagnosis.

Dr. Mayra later told me in an interview that she was inspired to adapt to her patients' "social realities" both by the training course and by her wider years of experience working in rural areas. As she explained,

> Because despite the fact that we are doctors, I think that we have to adapt. For example, with people who are profesionales, you can speak more calmly, in words that are a bit more, how can I say—it's not the

same to tell the señoras—for example, the señoras don't understand when you tell them, "Señora, *acuestese* [recline]." "What?" "Señora, *echate* [lie back]." In simpler words, no? That is, we as doctors cannot just say, "I only treat people from the city, not the country." So, if you treat people from the country, you have to adapt to them, speak in their language, speak like them. You can't say, "Señora, put yourself in a ventral position." She won't understand. [Instead, you have to say,] "On your *pancita* [little tummy], señora, lie down on your *barriguita* [little stomach]." I, as a doctor, won't attend a patient of just one social class—of just one type. There will always be a variety—poor, rich, foreign, native. Here we attend everyone.

Dr. Mayra framed her use of language both as an act of kindness and as a sign of her commitment to treating patients of different backgrounds. Echoing the skit she and other doctors had performed, she emphasized the importance of speaking gently (rather than harshly) and treating all patients equally. Like Dr. César, who had referenced legacies of colonialism, Dr. Mayra took up elements of state discourse in reflecting on how to engage difference in the medical setting and provide good care. She especially placed emphasis on the need to show kindness and pay attention to patients' social circumstances—in contrast to the forms of scolding that were still common practice in the hospital. Yet while she did not engage in the forms of chastisement I described earlier in this chapter, a warmer approach remained entangled in enduring dynamics of racialization and medical paternalism that had become naturalized in the clinic. The use of the diminutive "-ita" at the end of words (panc*ita*, barrigu*ita*) was common in Bolivian Spanish; it carried valences of familiarity and closeness. However, in combination with the use of simpler language and the informal second person (echa*te*, instead of the more formal acueste*se*), the diminutive positioned patients as childlike, as not capable of full reasoning.

Dr. Mayra could not be certain what Leonardo had. Omeprazole reduced stomach acidity, but she did not have the tools at her disposal to determine, for example, the underlying microbial cause. Instead, pressing on the abdomen became the best way of understanding pain. Yet within this space of uncertainty—where Dr. Mayra also had to assert her own experience and judgment to make care work—she also continued to locate a barrier to her practice within Leonardo himself.

The communicative injustices (Briggs and Mantini Briggs 2016) that long characterized Bolivian medical encounters were arguably reinscribed in new forms under the promise of warmth, inclusion, and cariño. Dr. Mayra hoped to do good for patients, emphasizing the importance of adapting to context and attending to what she saw as patient needs; warmth combined the language of attention with that of liberal equality and inclusion. Yet both modes of care continued to rely on the same underlying presuppositions of racial, linguistic, and embodied difference. Dr. Mayra read Leonardo, an Aymara speaker, as less capable of understanding complex medical processes and diagnoses—and rural Aymara patients more broadly as needing to be addressed in simplified language.[7] Here, the working assumption continued to be, "They don't understand me," rather than the reverse of, "I don't understand them." Aymara phrases, diminutive language, and gestures became, in Mayra's view, a way to communicate medical information on a level she assumed he would understand.

Patients themselves sometimes described demonstrations of warmth from providers in positive terms—as shows of cariño could index providers' greater attentiveness and investment in patients. Often, however, patients placed emphasis not just on shows of fleeting kindness, but on providers spending time with patients and, very often, coming to a satisfactory diagnosis. A handful of doctors who had lived and worked in Machacamarca for years and had built up relationships with town residents were especially well regarded. Dr. Mauricio, who had worked in the hospital for ten years, was often criticized by other doctors for taking up too much time with his appointments, therefore creating a backlog of patients, but patients frequently praised him and called him on the phone whenever they had a medical concern. Dr. Ignacio, who administered the Bono Juana Azurduy (the subsidy for pre- and post-natal care) was from Machacamarca originally and had returned to work there; thus he was also well known in town. Patients affectionately (and quite humorously) nicknamed him "Dr. Bonito," a play on the word "Bono" (*Bono* means subsidy, but *bonito* means "nice" or "pretty"). When built into more substantial relations, the cariño doctors showed toward patients could also be returned with patients' own cariño toward them.

But warmth could be tenuous—and especially in a context of uncertainty and resource shortages, patients hoped that providers might be able to grant a clear authoritative diagnosis. Doing so could be challenging for doctors who themselves were navigating material uncertainty. At the same time, echoing Dr. Mayra's approach with Leonardo, doctors frequently declined to explain diagnoses and simply handed patients a prescription to take to the pharmacy, on the assumption patients would not fully understand all of the details of their condition. However, in the waiting room I often ran into patients asking providers they trusted to explain a diagnosis or prescription to them, in the hopes that it would grant them some certainty. In one instance, a patient stopped Dr. Mauricio to show him the prescription another hospital doctor had provided and ask him what it was for. In another, a patient with a broken wrist asked Lucinda, one of the hospital's parteras, to help her interpret an X ray of her wrist because the biomedical provider who had taken the X ray had not done so. Lucinda was not trained in biomedicine but did work as a *naturista* (natural healer), and the patient trusted her to point out the fracture on the X ray.

Most often, however, patients were concerned about inattention and abandonment from doctors—a dynamic that patients sometimes described as "cold" in ways that were not always sufficiently countered by fleeting moves toward warm care. I met Valerio when he was hospitalized for several days to treat a burn. The hospital, centered as it was on primary and emergency care, rarely housed more than a few patients at a time for longer stays. He was alone in one of the small overnight rooms in the back of the building. He sat on the edge of the white plastic bed, surrounded by a tangle of faded sheets, his aged shoulders hunched forward. An oxygen mask covered the lower half of his face, linking him through a long thin tube to a dark green cylinder.

I asked him, cautiously, if he felt well enough to talk. He nodded and began speaking in a rambling rush, pausing only to draw long, rattling breaths through the oxygen mask. It was as if he had latched onto me as a willing listener in an otherwise empty room. He recounted,

> I burned my foot with fire. And in the hospital, they said, "Now, you will be cured." But I am here without a sweater. They are making me suffer. They are making me catch a cold. This is how I am feeling right now. . . . They will arrive late. Maybe they will arrive, or maybe they will not arrive. I will have to wait until late for sure. . . . What will they say? How will it be now? . . . And about these medications, what will they say? I am just waiting. Will they cure me, or not? I still don't know, really, if they will cure me. If they don't, then that's how it is.

In Valerio's recounting, the cold hospital temperature intersected with cold neglect of being left alone, and of the uncertainty that the medications he would be given would even work. Yet the kinds of more substantial material and ethical investments that Valerio and others hoped for were also made difficult by the working conditions of the hospital itself, as providers were overburdened with other tasks and could not come in regularly to check up on patients staying in long-term care, and as the pharmacy did not always have available medications. In this context, providers' acts of warm care—such as a phrase in Aymara, or softer and more diminutive words—could potentially index deeper attention from providers if followed up with other actions. But it did not always lead to remedying the problems that might make patients feel cold.

Yet for providers (and for those who administered policy and designed training courses) warm care was often a concrete and feasible way to transform their care for the better, when discussions of colonialism and capitalism in the textbook (in their view) remained abstract. But much like the forms of chastisement that also continued to persist as care in the hospital, it reentrenched hierarchies in the hospital and deflected from the conditions that produced them.

In interviews, policymakers based in La Paz frequently expressed to me that the most substantial barrier to transforming health care was biomedical practitioners, whom they described as resistant to change. In framing barriers in this way, they echoed the language of blame that also circulated among biomedical practitioners. Sometimes, practitioners blamed each other (with Cuban-trained and Bolivian-trained doctors pitted against one another). But they especially blamed patients.

Blame, as I came to understand it, came from a place of frustration with constrained circumstances—frustration with the inability to enact the policy change one had envisioned, or frustration with the inability to cure patients and provide the biomedical care one hoped for. In contrast to other vocal forms of frustration like complaint that I return to later in the book (see Chapter 6), blame often involved shifting frustrations onto those with comparatively less power. Structural violence, I suggest, created the obfuscations that led to shifting blame onto individuals.

And yet, it was the broader social and material structures that were central to the endurance of inequality in the clinic. Enduring racialized modes of intervention were not a problem of individual mentality that could be workshopped away, or that might be mitigated with urges to be kinder. Instead, they reflected how habituated modes of care remained tied to wider social structures of race and class hierarchy as well as the material redistribution of resources.

For many providers, the training course became an idealized site of moral imagination, where they could ponder and act out how care might be or should be. But in situating structural inequalities primarily in the past and in the abstract, the course did not ask practitioners to engage with the everyday ways that social inequality and resource constraints continued to profoundly shape their own world and that of their patients. Inequalities continued to be reinscribed in the ordinary practice of the clinic—not only despite state pushes to adopt care "with quality and warmth," but also with and through warm care. Training course efforts to encourage practitioners to be warmer and more affectionate were discursively tied to combatting discrimination and treating all patients equally. Yet moves toward warmth relied on—and continued to reproduce—long-standing racializing presuppositions, enacted through routinized forms of clinical care for Indigenous and low-income patients.

3 WARM AND COLD

Cultural Adaptation and the Circulation of Temperature

THE "CULTURALLY ADAPTED" BIRTHING ROOM (*sala con adecuación cultural*) of the Machacamarca Hospital at first glance appeared out of place—a respite from the severe white tiles and walls that spread through most of the hospital. In the culturally adapted room, the floors and wooden walls were a deep, terra-cotta orange. Instead of a gynecological gurney, there were two wooden beds, draped in woolen blankets, decorated with printed blankets. Faded posters, describing the different birthing positions one might use, hung crookedly on the walls. In the corner, a portable gas stove perched on the counter next to the sink. Pots, pans, tin cups, and soup bowls were displayed inside a locked glass cabinet, while medical supplies were hidden from sight inside a wooden chest of drawers. And the room was warm. The sturdy construction buffered the cold winds that blew through the rest of the building, creating a sheltered enclave (Figure 3.1).

The space was a stark contrast to the older, laboratory-like birthing room just down the hall. Still used for emergencies and high-risk births, the older room had a white-tiled floor and white painted walls. A spindly metal gurney and dark green oxygen tank sat in the middle of the room, lit from overhead with harsh fluorescent lighting. White

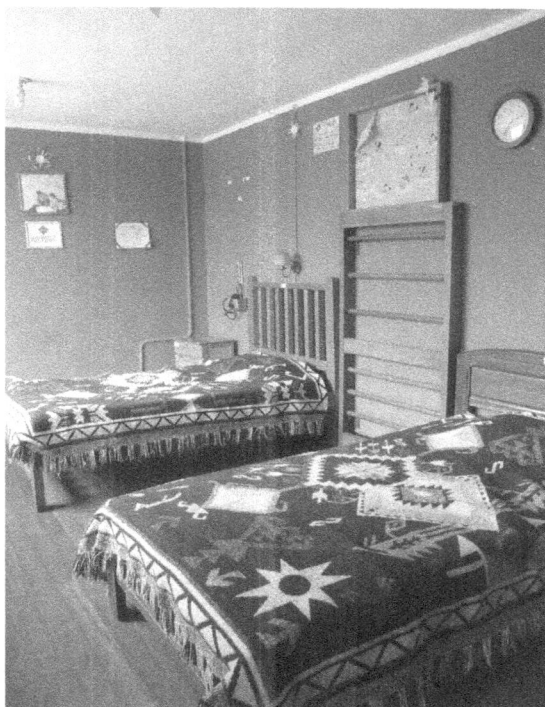

FIGURE 3.1. The culturally adapted birthing room in the Machacamarca Hospital. Source: Photograph by the author.

counters and shelves displayed medical supplies. The tile floors and thin walls allowed the cold Altiplano air to seep in (Figure 3.2).

In 2008, GHA constructed the Machacamarca Hospital's first culturally adapted birthing room. It constructed two additional rooms in 2011. NGO workers, as well as Bolivian state officials, suggested that the new rooms would create conditions for a more comfortable birthing experience for Aymara women, many of whom preferred to give birth at home. They indicated that, in the culturally adapted room, women could give birth in the company of a family member and a midwife. Although not an exact reproduction, the room was designed to evoke the familiar environment of Aymara women's homes.

Continuing the discussion begun in Chapter 2, this chapter exam-

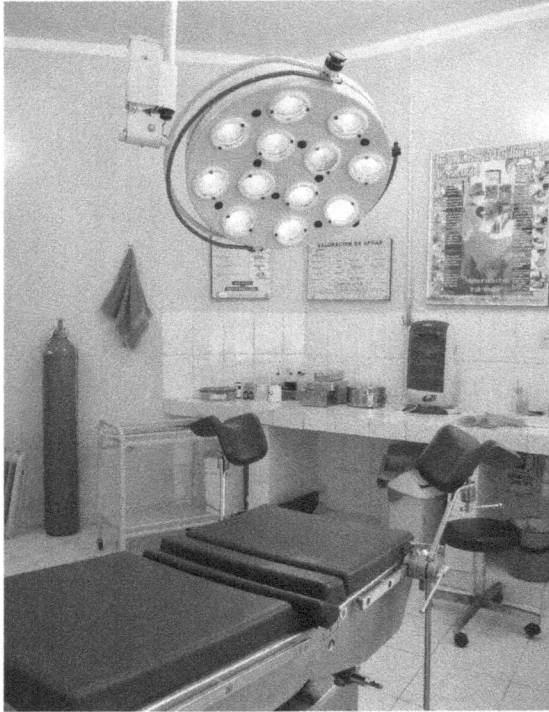

FIGURE 3.2. The laboratory-like birthing room in the Machacamarca Hospital. Source: Photograph by the author.

ines another effort to reorient biomedical care—this time, through the construction of culturally adapted birthing rooms. Although constructed by a transnationally funded NGO, the culturally adapted birthing rooms were taken up by state officials, biomedical practitioners, and even NGO workers themselves as a key component of the state's project to move toward a decolonized and intercultural health care system. As I heard a doctor remark to a woman going into labor at the hospital, "It is thanks to Evo that you can give birth in a room like this." In this chapter, I examine how the material space of the home—historically a site of biopolitical concern about gendered Indigenous "cultural" threats to life—was invoked, imitated, and remade in the hospital context in the name of extending recognition.

Specifically, I examine how temperature (as an ontological, material, and sensorial element) became central to efforts to make the hospital space more home-like. Attention to temperature as a site of ethnographic analysis obliges us to consider how the warm care of Bolivian institutional decolonizing projects entailed not only a shift in affective dispositions but also a reworking of material elements that came to bear on the body. In the context of home births, residents of Machacamarca attended to the cold as a lively, potentially dangerous force that could cause sickness or death of the laboring mother. Yet in the context of the hospital birthing rooms, institutional actors enacted warmth not as a matter of life and death, but in terms of invitation and "psychological support." I show how in the culturally adapted birthing room, physical and sensorial architectural projects were intimately tied to the state's warm care—and specifically, to its promise of inclusivity and good feeling for Indigenous patients.

I also examine how the reworking of temperature between home and hospital enabled some formations of care while foreclosing others. STS scholars Jeannette Pols and Ingunn Moser (2009) have compellingly challenged perceived divisions between "cold technologies and warm care." They argue that, far from being separate from or antithetical to care, medical technologies often deemed "cold" are in fact central to constituting affectively warm social relations in the clinic. While I agree with their broader challenge to perceived distinctions between care and technology, I consider how medical technologies specifically designed with warmth in mind also generate particular moral and material practices in the clinic. I argue that while the clinical mobilization of warm matter and practice at times enabled new forms of intimate care during hospital birth, it also extended racializing logics that positioned culture as a threat to be managed.

TEMPERATURE AS LIVELY FORCE

At roughly 3,800 meters (or approximately 12,500 feet) above sea level, the Bolivian Altiplano was cold much of the year. In the dry and sunny winters, temperatures dropped to below freezing, and winds blew across the plains that cut the bone like a knife. The summer months brought occasional relief, with light rains and temperatures rising to a medium-cool. As I learned from many of my interlocutors, knowing how to be in the cold—and live well in the cold—required continual attention to how external influences could come to bear on health and illness, life and death. In predominantly Aymara and Quechua communities in the Bolivian Andes, it was well known that bodily states could be influenced by many exogenous forces: extreme temperatures, but also social relations, emotions, and the histories of places (Canessa 2012; Crandon-Malamud 1991; Tapias 2015). Bodily ontologies were iterated through deep histories of colonization—as, much like across the Latin American continent, humoral theories of bodily equilibrium and malleability, imposed through Iberian colonization and missionary teachings, were rerouted and renegotiated through existing Indigenous relational practices (Koss-Chioino, Leatherman, and Greenway 2003; Sanabria 2016). During childbirth, the body was porous and vulnerable to outside influences, especially those of temperature; cold entering the body could cause severe illness, even death (Loza and Álvarez Quispe 2011). Thus, when a woman gave birth at home, caregivers paid special attention to helping her maintain a warm bodily state.

As I learned from conversations with people who had either given birth at home or helped others give birth at home, home births were an intimate practice, often with only close family members present. During birth, the husband especially was expected to take on a central role of keeping his wife's body warm by preparing hot teas and soups, heating fires, and giving massages that would help her maintain a bodily equilibrium and protect her body from the cold. The wife's mother or mother-in-law frequently stepped in to assist as well. Family members might in addition call upon the help of a *yatiri* (ritual healer) or midwife (*partera* in Spanish, *usuyiri* in Aymara). They did so especially when the husband lacked experience or could not be present, or when a complication arose that the family could not resolve (Arnold and Yapita 2002; Canessa 2012; Loza and Álvarez Quispe 2011; Platt 2013). Many parteras were family or community members with a reputation for being knowledgeable, and some of them were also supernaturally marked with the gift of healing. They drew on extensive apprenticed and experiential knowledge, including how to read pulses to time the birth, prepare herbal teas, and, if needed, adjust the position of the fetus (Arnold and Yapita 2002; UNFPA 2012).

Providing care during childbirth involved both skill and experience attuning to temperature and other forces that might act on the body. Many husbands I interviewed spoke with pride of their knowledge and skill, describing how they had provided good care so that their wives did not suffer.[1] My elderly neighbor Augusto had been the primary caregiver for his wife, Modesta, for the births of each of their five children. He described to me how he knew which plants to gather to make hot teas and prepare fortifying soups (with mutton, no spice) to keep his wife warm before, during, and after labor.

Once, however, after the birth of their youngest daughter, Modesta developed *sobreparto*. An illness etiology common in the rural Andes, although not always recognized in the biomedical context, sobreparto involved coagulation of the blood inside the abdomen as a result of exposure to extreme temperatures during and after birth and manifested in fever, cold, sweat, and chills. It often rendered a woman unable to care for her newborn—and could lead to her death.[2] Augusto emphasized the careful, material work he undertook to heal his wife:

> I prepared her a remedy for sobreparto in the sun. We prepared a *waja* [a method of cooking with a fire lit under a small mound of soil and rocks] where the soil was red. Everything was scorched. There is red soil like that from the sun, in the grass plains. Also, the firewood has been left out in the sun for a long time. The wood stopped being fresh years ago. So, one has to gather the dry wood. One has to gather it in the sun. And some rocks, too—they should be nice and hot. One has to put everything there, put the rocks in place. But one should not touch them with the hands, but with a spoon, to move them. One to three rocks, like that. And bring the liquid almost to a boil, making a foam. And then she has to drink it. Drink it and sleep. This is a medicine from the sun. Usually, when one has taken too much sun, one is weak. But when one has just given birth, it is good. Then she has to sweat. One has to sweat it out when one has caught a cold.

Augusto's didactic narrative—switching seamlessly from a description of what he did in a specific instance to a more general discussion of how one should address sobreparto—pointed to how care required practiced skill and attention to how temperature affected the body. Yet his perspective was subject to some debate. Another neighbor, Andrés, suggested that too much sun could, in fact, also bring on sobreparto. As he suggested, "Cold brings sickness. So does the sun. So, one has to take care of her—for one month if the baby is a boy and three weeks if the baby is a girl. This is how we take care of ourselves. This is how I take care of my wife." He described how, in addition to preparing soups and teas, he would help her take a warm, rosemary-infused bath and then rub her with animal fat to protect her from the cold. "Our skin is full of small holes—they are called 'pores,' right? So that is why she has to be well covered. Otherwise, it's open, and she can get sick." Although the two men disagreed on the best techniques of care, both tinkered with tangible technologies—teas, blankets, fires, stoves, baths, fat—that had the capacity to warm. For both, care also involved attention to elements of climate and air, as temperature flowed through space and bodies.

Pushing back against dominant biomedical narratives in Bolivia that sobreparto is not real—or that it is just another way of describing postpartum infection—traditional medicine scholars Carmen Beatriz Loza and Walter Álvarez Quispe (2011) call for taking sobreparto seriously as an embodied set of symptoms, central to Aymara knowledge about childbirth. In a similar vein, medical anthropologists have traced embodied experiences of sobreparto as they relate to situated knowledges and social worlds (Crandon-Malamud 1991; Guerra-Reyes 2019; Larme and Leatherman 2003). Karolina Kuberska (2016), for example, has suggested that experiences of sobreparto among Aymara women who have migrated to the lowland city of Santa Cruz emerge at the nexus of social distress, loneliness, and being insufficiently cared for. Building on these perspectives, I suggest that Augusto's and Andrés's narratives also point to how moral questions of care were inseparable from material ontologies, including how temperature acted on the body.

Indigenous Studies scholars have long highlighted the centrality of relations with other-than-human entities in constituting worlds (de la Cadena 2015; Hokowhitu 2020; Todd 2016; Watts 2013)—a concern that has likewise been taken up in STS research with increased attention to the vibrancy of matter, as it both constitutes and exceeds human interaction (Bennet 2010; Barad 2003).[3] These perspectives affirm how, in the practice of care, persons, bodies, and material technologies are continually brought into relation (Mol 2008; Mol, Moser, and Pols 2015). To put it differently, moral practice is not separate from the material but co-constitutive with it. Temperature was a vibrant force that one had to engage with and be attentive to; it was inseparable from questions of human relations and showing proper care and attention.

These dynamics—of good care being tied to material relations—were especially reflected in gendered ways of recounting the work of childbirth. Many men I interviewed boasted of their knowledge and skill, describing to me how they had provided good care so that their wife did not suffer. Echoing the findings of Tristan Platt (2013), who likewise takes note of gendered ways of talking about birth, women often shared more variable perspectives. Many did not go into detail about their experiences of birth at all, while others commented on whether their husbands had been sufficiently attentive. In these instances, skilled and attentive work—rooted in part in attunement to temperature—became central to notions of what it was to provide good care (or when it failed to be enacted).

These moral and material fields of care were also brought unevenly to bear on engagements with hospital-based births. The hospital was—in more ways than one—a cold space. In private clinics in the cities, husbands were usually allowed to enter the room during birth, and doctors provided their patients with personalized attention. But in public institutions like the Machacamarca Hospital, patients frequently described treatment as impersonal as well as uncertain. When a woman came to the hospital in labor, the doctor who happened to be on shift in the emergency room delivered the baby—so patients and practitioners were often meeting for the first time. In the laboratory-like birthing room, practitioners refused entry to family members, including the husband. To give birth, patients lay on the gynecological gurney; it was a narrow, old-fashioned apparatus—the kind one no longer saw in more well-to-do-clinics—with a rigid plastic cushion and a stirrup that wiggled loose, so that sometimes the nurse had to hold it in place while the patient gave birth. Most patients claimed it was uncomfortable, cold, and creaky. Doctors' and nurses' movements and tones of voice were, at times, brusque. For at least some medical practitioners, harshness and scolding were necessary to good care practice in a context in which resources were few and patients were deemed noncompliant (see Chapter 2). When a birth did not come easily, they told their patients that they were not pushing or breathing correctly, or that they were not trying hard enough. Cold materials and cold affects were closely intertwined.

Yet if many women I spoke to were critical of the hospital and described it as a cold space, they did not disengage completely from the hospital. With increased availability of biomedicine that had not been present a generation ago, as well as increased rural-to-urban migration, modes of giving birth were also changing. Most (although not all) women under thirty who I interviewed had given birth in the Machacamarca Hospital or their local health center, while most (although not all) older women had given birth at home. Some women had also changed the way they gave birth over time; if they had given birth to their eldest children at home, they had given birth to their younger children in the hospital. Rosa, who was in her late thirties, had given birth to her older son at home, with the help of her husband and mother, in the village where she lived at the time. It had been a difficult birth, and she could not get pregnant for many years afterwards. Ten years later, she moved with her family to the town of Machacamarca, and she got pregnant again. As she later recounted, older kin (los viejitos) had told her she should give birth in the hospital, because they could tell that the fetus was badly positioned in her womb. Recalling other accounts I had heard, I asked her if her older kin had suggested shifting the position of the fetus using a cloth wrap (a technique called manteo that some older women knew how to do). She replied that no, they had advised her to go to the hospital because her pregnancy was "not normal."

Notions of the "normal birth" (*parto normal*) had increasingly worked their way into and alongside other practices that centered on caring for the porous and humoral body—and shaped the plural ways that women understood their own bodies and assessed the risks of pregnancy. That is, amid the persistence of cold in the hospital and ongoing ambivalence of care, women and their families would weigh various factors. Ontologies of the body, rather than culturally fixed, were continually recontextualized—or as Emilia Sanabria suggests, were "actively recombined in ways that both transform and allow them to endure in new forms" (2016, 53).

In this shifting medical context, for example, some women with whom I spoke preferred to come to the hospital only for prenatal exams to assure themselves that everything was "normal" before giving birth at home. One morning in the hospital, I met a young couple, Laura and Roberto, who had come to the hospital multiple times to get an ultrasound, just to check that the pregnancy was normal, but they planned to have a home birth. But each time they had come, the ultrasound technician was unavailable because of staffing shortages. The last time they came—on the morning I met them—the primary care doctor informed Laura that she was already in labor, and that they would have to move her to the laboratory-like birthing room because the fetus was premature. The next day, I spoke again with Laura, as she was resting with her newborn. She had not thought she would give birth in the hospital, she complained. All her previous births had been at home, with the help of a partera, and she had only come to the hospital to determine if there would be any complications. "But I came in vain," she said. "Because when I came, there was no ultrasound."

LETTING THE HOME INTO THE HOSPITAL

Before working as the field director for GHA, Alicia had been employed in the late 1990s and early 2000s at a Bolivian NGO in Potosí called Kawsay (a pseudonym) that was one of the first to experiment with adapting health centers to incorporate some elements of home births. The NGO developed guidelines that would later provide the basis for state policies under Evo Morales as well as GHA's work constructing birthing rooms in Machacamarca and surrounding areas. As Alicia explained, one of Kawsay's central missions was to bring down high maternal-infant mortality rates in the Bolivian countryside. She described to me how she came to understand maternal mortality as a pressing concern because of her own experiences being placed in a small rural health center through her work with the NGO. As she explained, one particular incident forever shaped her outlook. I reproduce her narrative in its entirety below:

> Maternal mortality was really high. I was there; I saw it for myself. One time, I was working in the health center. In the evening someone called to say that "Señora Such-and-Such had her baby at home yesterday and now she is hemorrhaging."
>
> The auxiliary nurse [who answered the phone] asked, "Is there abundant hemorrhaging? How is it? There is just a little?"
>
> "Yes, just a little."
>
> "Okay. Tell the señora to stay. It is nighttime, and we cannot go. It is dangerous" [the auxiliary nurse said]. Because you see, we had to go far, over rough terrain, crossing rivers. "Tell the señora to please rest, to drink lots of fluids."
>
> At the time, we were not too worried, because they said there was only a little hemorrhaging. I heard the health personnel say, "They said the señora is hemorrhaging, but maybe it's not the case. Because when I asked, they said it was not abundant. They said there was very little. So, tomorrow we can leave very early and arrive at her house in daylight."
>
> But when we arrived the next day, the señora had died. Something else happened—I am trying to remember. I think our truck had also broken down. I remember that there were many problems because of the rains, and we needed the truck to cross the rivers. What happened was that night she began having a more massive hemorrhage, and when we arrived she had already entered into hypovolemic shock. She died because she bled out. So, it was very bad. The health person-

nel should have gone. The truck was broken down but they should have
gone on foot, even at night.

After that moment, I developed an even greater commitment to
working on the problem of maternal mortality. That is, I wanted to
know: Why hadn't the señora come to the health center, so that the
health personnel could treat her? And then the study we did brought us
to propose strategies of working with parteras and adapting the space.
That is, the establishment was cold, so we needed to think about what
we could do.

Alicia's voice trembled as she told this story, still affected decades
later by the injustice of a death that could have been prevented. She
was ready to allocate responsibility for the woman's death across multiple sites, including the material factors limiting the health center
staff's capacity to provide timely care (the rough terrain, the broken-
down truck) as well as the provider's hesitation and, perhaps, unwill-
ingness to take the patient seriously ("just a little bleeding"). Yet by the
end of the tale, she ultimately turned to emphasizing the question of
why the woman herself had not gone to the health center. Rather than
asking whether the patient might also face challenges of lack of transport or traveling over rough terrain, Alicia focused on the woman's
possible lack of willingness to come because "the establishment was
cold"—which might be addressed through "working with parteras and
adapting the space."

Tackling these problems of cold was precisely what Kawsay ended
up doing. The organization hired a team of anthropologists and sociologists to determine why mostly Quechua women living in Potosí's rural regions were not coming to health centers to give birth.
According to Alicia, their studies concluded that many were afraid
because the building was cold, and they might develop sobreparto
as a result. Based on their findings, the Kawsay team recommended
building warmer spaces in the health center. Alicia described how
they translated their research into what became known as a culturally adapted space:

The women didn't really analyze it, but we heard them say that they wanted the space to be warmer. I remember that the birthing rooms had tile, and when you entered it was terribly cold. And they said, "No, I am going to get sobreparto." There were also other factors. There was fear of the health personnel, distrust. "The doctor won't understand me, what I need. Moreover, I need the company of my husband, my mother, and the partera." The other issue was the physical conditions of the space. They needed an equilibrium between cold and hot. They did not want anything metallic, because it was cold. They said, "There can't be tiles." And so, they said, "What can we put? Bricks." So, the floor was brick, because brick is warmer. Later, we began analyzing that they, for example, generally gave birth in the kitchen, because it was warmer. So, we put in a kitchen.

These NGO findings resonated with wider anthropological findings about the central role of temperature in childbirth in the Andes—as well as my own conversations with families in Machacamarca. As NGOs and other transnational development organizations have increasingly come to center questions of cultural difference in their work, their approaches draw from and overlap with anthropological categories and methods. At the same time, they also embrace different framings that translate culture into a fixed and tangible site of policy intervention. Tania Li calls for attention to how development organizations gather data to "render technical" local communities and practices as sites of intervention; in doing so, they "identif[y] an area of intervention, [bind] it, [dissect] it, and [devise] corrective measures to produce desirable results" (2007, 123). As Li argues, in narrowly defining conditions as "technical problems" with "technical solutions," organizations can also miss or ignore the wider social, political, and economic circumstances that policy recipients face.

My conversations with NGO and state actors suggested that the study and subsequent interventions reframed temperature (a lively force in the context of home births) as a technical problem of managing "cultural barriers" (barreras culturales), understood to be the primary contributor to maternal-infant mortality, to the exclusion of other material and structural factors. In this context, temperature also took a new form: a means to provide what many described as a form of "psychological support" (*apoyo psicológico*) for patients during childbirth. More easily legible to institutional actors, more easily commensurate with hospital-based care, the paradigm of "psychological support" rerouted warmth from a potent agent of bodily well-being to a technology for calming patients and quelling their fears. Though imbued with good intentions and feelings—discursively centered on the need to provide Indigenous patients with a better birthing experience—it carried echoes of earlier presuppositions: that cultural difference (as code for race) explained patients' fundamental fear of biomedicine, that they needed to be urged to "collaborate" (see Chapter 2). Now, however, the goal was to offer a modicum of comfort to bring patients into the hospital—primarily through the adjusting of material elements and space.

The idea to resolve cultural barriers by making birthing rooms more "home-like" echoed broader regional trends. Across numerous Latin American contexts, national and regional governments (often with substantial support from NGOs and global health agencies) have sought since the 1990s to adopt intercultural health policies, framed in terms of making biomedicine more inclusive of Indigenous patients' cultural practices. Especially when it came to childbirth, such policies often involved a transformation of the hospital space itself, so that the paradigmatic referent shifted from the laboratory to the home. Initiatives ranged, for example, from installing hammocks in a hospital in the Mexican state of Campeche (Campos Navarro et al 1997; Vega 2018), to incorporating squatting chairs and radiators in clinics near Cusco, Peru (Guerra-Reyes 2019), and, in highland Bolivia, to building warm, orange-hued rooms with beds and small kitchens. While resonant with recent moves to create more "humanized" and "patient-centered" hospital spaces around the globe (Bates 2018), these architectural initiatives were specifically couched in terms of recognizing cultural difference—and thereby reducing maternal mortality by bringing more patients into the hospital.

Building on the prior work undertaken by NGOs like Kawsay, GHA staffers developed models that they frequently suggested were authentically Indigenous; they insisted that their models were not like prior NGO interventions that "hung up *aguayos* (colorful woven cloths) and called it 'cultural adaptation.'" Yet authenticity in construction stemmed less from exact replication of people's home environments than from the affects that these materials enabled. None of the homes I entered in Machacamarca and its surrounding areas had terra-cotta colored walls; they ranged from unpainted mud-brick to concrete walls painted in white, blue, green, and yellow. When I asked GHA staffers why they had chosen the orange color, they often referred to a study conducted years prior stating that patients preferred warm colors. Alicia also explained that some home conditions (like sheep-skins on the floor or fires that families burned) would be unhygienic in the hospital setting. As Elizabeth Povinelli (2002) notes, the logics of cultural recognition require that Indigenous peoples perform au-thentic cultural difference, but only on terms that settlers do not find repugnant (or in this case, do not find threatening to life and to bio-medical intervention). Instead, authenticity derived from the room's warmth (*calidez*) and its articulation of Indigenous understandings of a hot-cold equilibrium. Warmth was rendered in stylized terms; the room appeared almost museum-like with its terra-cotta walls, printed blankets, and glass cabinets that displayed cups and bowls but were never unlocked because, according to hospital staff, patients would steal items.

The idea that warm architectures might simultaneously reflect Indigenous patients' authentic cultural experience and help address their supposed cultural resistance to biomedical care also percolated out to other sites—and other material technologies. A Bolivian Ministry of Health publication on implementing culturally adapted maternal health protocols, for example, stated the following: "When possible, one must try to avoid dressing in a white coat, hair covering, or mask. One also cannot require those who accompany the woman in labor to wear shoe coverings or a mask" (Ministerio de Salud y Deportes 2006, 22, my translation). Next to the guideline was the crossed-out image of doctors wearing full protective gear. In the margins, a small cartoon figure stated in a word bubble, "We should not wear white clothing, because the Indigenous patients do not like it. One also should not use white sheets on the bed, because the women are afraid of making them dirty" (Ministerio de Salud y Deportes 2006, 22, my translation).

For Lucía Guerra-Reyes, writing on intercultural birthing policies in neighboring Peru, a key limitation of such policies is that while they reflect institutional efforts to engage Indigenous birthing practices, "these practices have been cherry-picked and divorced from the cultural systems in which they have meaning" (2019, 7). Living in Machacamarca, I encountered no one who expressed fear of light colors or of medical outfits, although some residents expressed fear of going to the hospital in general. They described how "people just go to the hospital to die" and expressed concerns about resource shortages in the hospital and mistreatment from doctors. Yet, in its guidebook, the Ministry of Health reframed patient concerns about the conditions of public hospitals and clinics into a much narrower fear of white coats and sheets that Indigenous patients inherently "do not like." Ministry and NGO officials echoed older narratives that placed Indigenous women's inability to become modern subjects with their traditions. It relied on an implicit comparison: that white and mestizo citizens, living in urban areas, already knew how to give birth and did not need to be coaxed into medical spaces as Indigenous peoples did.

Institutional preoccupations with invoking the home environment and coaxing presumably reluctant patients into the hospital were central to emergent forms of warm care in Bolivia. Officials expressed deep concern with making patients feel included and "at home"—even as they relied on long-standing racial stereotypes and narratives of institutional benevolence to do so. As Dian Million (2013) and Audra Simpson (2020) argue, settler discourses of humanitarian sympathy and good feeling can often be deployed in ways that depoliticize Indigenous struggles and maintain ongoing structures of dispossession. In this context, temperature also mattered for care—but it mattered differently. It shifted from a dynamic force at the heart of kin-based moral practice to a technology that would presumably quell fears and offer psychological support during birth. As I will go on to show, this was also a perspective taken up—and renegotiated—by biomedical practitioners, who often weighed what kinds of warmth they could permit in the hospital.

DRAWING BOUNDARIES

The first two times Berta came to the hospital to give birth some years ago, the doctor gave her the option of using either the culturally adapted room or the biomedical room. She remembered it well, because this time no one asked which room she would prefer. The nurse brought her straight to the biomedical birthing room when she went into labor. Her husband, Ramiro, pulled the nurse aside. "It's cold in here," he said. "Can't she be in the other room?"

The nurse, Ximena, looked at the forms. "Is this her first birth?" she asked.

Ramiro shook his head. "Her third."

Ximena hesitated briefly. "Then that should be fine. I'll let the doctor know." She pushed Berta in the wheelchair down the hall to the culturally adapted room. Ramiro helped Berta onto the bed, lifting the woolen blankets. Berta was heavy with contractions and looked like she would give birth any minute. Ximena quickly trotted out of the room and returned rolling a small metal cart full of medical supplies (clamps, eyedrops, disinfectant). I helped her spread a long, black tarp over the bed.

"Will you be staying?" the nurse asked Ramiro. He nodded.

We heard the door creak open, and Dr. Verónica entered. Walking over to the bed, she asked Ramiro to leave the room while she measured Berta's dilation so that Berta could have some privacy. The doctor sat on the edge of the bed to examine her patient. Suddenly, she announced the baby would be emerging any minute. She snatched up the bundle she had brought into the room—a green gown to drape over her scrubs, a net to pull tight over her hair, and a mask to stretch across the lower half of her face. By the time she had finished adjusting her many layers, she was barely recognizable underneath. She sat back down on the corner of the bed, at an angle, so that she could deliver the newborn when the time came.

There was a loud banging at the door. Ximena walked over and cracked it open. "It's the husband," she called back to Dr. Veronica. "He wants to come in. He says he has rights."

Dr. Verónica shook her head curtly. "No."

After the procedure, I stayed to talk with Ramiro and Berta and congratulate them on the birth of their son. Ramiro was livid that he had been kept out of the room, explaining that the first two times they had come to the hospital, the doctor on shift had allowed him to stay. Ramiro recounted how they had thought the room warmer and more comfortable than the rest of the hospital, which is why they asked to use it again. His words highlighted how the warmth of the room could still create conditions for a good birth, preferable to the conditions found in the other, more laboratory-like birthing room. Although not quite like the conditions of a home birth, some patients appreciated— and actively demanded—elements of care promised in the construction of the room, including the presence of family members, the use of a kitchen, and a more comfortable bed. In this instance, when these promises were denied, Ramiro sought to push back and claim what he described as his rights as the spouse.

In the laboratory-like birthing room, it was common to make family members wait on the other side of a bright red line painted across the floor, right outside the door. Doctors argued that family members were often anxious or wanted to interfere, making obstetric practice more difficult. By keeping Ramiro out—even when the protocols of cultural adaptation required that he stay—Dr. Verónica sought to mirror the practices she was accustomed to enacting in the biomedical birthing room. As she explained, the culturally adapted room was unhygienic and potentially dangerous, so she sought to transform it into a safer, more controlled environment. Many of the general medical practitioners working in the hospital expressed views similar to Dr. Verónica's: that the culturally adapted room did not meet the standards of scientific intervention found in the laboratory-like room down the hall. Like Dr. Verónica, many sought to also reinscribe biomedical relations in the culturally adapted room—ultimately pushing back against the idea that Indigenous culture had any place in medicine at all.

Writing in the context of Guatemalan reproductive health care, Nicole Berry (2010) notes that globalized forms of biomedicine often center on treating the patient body as an autonomous entity, decontextualized from kin and other social relations that characterize home birthing. In Machacamarca, biomedical practitioners' desire to isolate the patient body took the form of physical control over the environment (like keeping family members out) as well as the treatment of the body in parts (exemplified in the laboratory-like birthing rooms by doctors draping sheets over the patient's legs, so that all parts of the patient except for the vaginal opening were hidden from view). While isolating and asserting medical authority over the patient body characterizes obstetric intervention in many contexts (Davis-Floyd 1992), in Bolivia these modes of intervention intersected in important ways with the class stratification of care and the racialization of Indigenous women's bodies. Middle- and upper-class mestiza women in urban centers in Bolivia could often access more personalized care and have their partners accompany them during birth; in contrast, practitioners in public clinics frequently treated Indigenous women as inherently unruly, as needing continual biomedical intervention and control. As I argued in Chapter 2, racialized presuppositions about patient bodies remained intact through policy efforts to encourage providers to adopt kindness and warmth in their practice. In the context of childbirth, these presuppositions underpinned authoritative modes of obstetric intervention, enacting what Dana-Aín Davis calls "obstetric racism" that emerges at the "intersection of obstetric violence and medical racism" (2019, 561).

In Machacamarca, control over the medical environment was tied to the racialization not only of patient bodies but also of others in the room, as physicians assessed who was interfering and who was not. While husbands like Ramiro were locked out, I was not, even though I was not a biomedical practitioner and could do nothing to aid in the birthing process. I sat in on several births in my time doing research in the hospital (and also interviewed countless others about their experiences afterwards). After receiving consent from patients and practitioners to be present, I usually tried to stay out of the way, although

I would sometimes help with minor tasks like rolling down a tarp on the bed or chatting to family members while waiting out contractions. I made it clear to all that I had no medical training. Yet, in contrast to their treatment of family members, physicians rarely considered me to be a potential interference. As a white woman imbued with the authority of a researcher, I was not construed as someone who would bring "culture" into the biomedical setting. These dynamics shaped how I accessed spaces as a researcher and highlighted how I was never far removed from the raced, classed, and gendered dynamics about which I was writing. They also point to how biomedical providers continually drew and redrew boundaries around what kinds of persons, bodies, relations, and temperatures could and could not enter the hospital.

As I came to better understand spending more time in the hospital, temperature mattered in different ways for providers at different points. Wearing puffy coats over their medical uniforms in the winter, biomedical practitioners frequently complained about their own discomfort in the cold hospital, as well as how temperature could have a negative impact on the provision of care. While hospitals needed to be kept cool to prevent the spread of bacteria, the freezing temperatures made some procedures more difficult. When undertaking minor surgeries, practitioners set up heat lamps in the room to bring the patient body to the correct temperature—but at the time of my research, only one of the three lamps the hospital had on hand was working. Cold temperatures were a constant source of preoccupation, as they often made it difficult to medically intervene in patient bodies.

Even so, many practitioners saw warm, culturally adapted objects and spaces as impeding their ability to provide the correct kind of care. Some time after I shadowed Dr. Verónica, I interviewed her about her work in the Machacamarca Hospital. She explained why delivering births in the culturally adapted room made her medical practice more difficult:

> For example, the beds should be set up with a tarp, so that the urine, the amniotic fluid, does not stain the bed. That should be set up before the patient enters, but it's not. They set it up right in the moment of

birth, and they set it up badly. So, there everything gets dirty, and it's uncomfortable for you, for the patient, for everyone really. What else is missing? There is no equipment to attend the neonate. The newborn. Nothing. And so, there, in the same bed as the mother. And I say that, for the moment, there haven't been any complications. At least in the shifts I was working, there were no complications, but in others' experiences, complications did present themselves. And so, for our safety, for us as well, I prefer to provide care in the biomedical room. . . . It's uncomfortable to provide care in the [culturally adapted] room. In the room, the patients don't open their legs, one can't properly do the curettage, one can't in the room. It was for that that they made gurneys.

From this perspective, warm matter in the culturally adapted room was not the right form to allow for proper intervention in patient bodies. According to Dr. Verónica, she could not maneuver the patient, or the emerging baby, correctly, and there was a constant risk of contamination. Culturally adapted technologies were too much like a home, and not enough like a hospital. So, while the space was designed with the idea of patient comfort in mind, it was decidedly uncomfortable for many general medical practitioners—revealing how they themselves were culturally attuned to the conditions of the biomedical birthing room.

Physicians contrived various strategies to mitigate what they perceived to be the dangers of the culturally adapted room. Although the protocols required that they give patients the choice to use the culturally adapted room, many of them found ways to use the laboratory-like room down the hall instead. They would use the culturally adapted room as a space where women could labor, and then transfer them down the hall when they were ready to give birth. Sometimes, however, doctors did use the room—perhaps because a patient demanded it or because NGO staffers were present that day. For doctors who were resistant to the idea, care work in the room required pragmatic renegotiations and reproducing the bodily affects and practices to which they were accustomed. Some kept family members—or even the hospital-sanctioned midwife—out. They used the same rough movements as in the other room—even as they had to angle themselves differently on the bed. Others brought in materials like the hospital gown from the other room. In short, they sought to reestablish the culturally adapted space as a hospital space where they could enact what they deemed to be appropriate forms of care.

RECOGNITION AND THE PSYCHOLOGY OF WARMTH

Yet even if most doctors argued that cultural adaptation made the practice of biomedicine difficult, a handful became advocates of using the room, articulating a different, although adjacent, notion of what constituted good care. Most of them had worked in the hospital for many years and participated in numerous workshops with the GHA and the Departmental Health Service on interculturality. Unlike their colleagues, they embraced the official argument that cultural adaptation could save patient lives by making women feel more comfortable and at home.

Dr. Edwin was a middle-aged practitioner with gray-streaked hair and a deep voice. He had been working in the hospital since before the first culturally adapted rooms were constructed, and he had become a strong advocate after taking a course at the Departmental Health Service. He complained the rooms had fallen out of use, and he frequently corrected other doctors he thought were using them improperly. He invited me to observe him as he worked, so that I could have an example of a correct culturally adapted birth for my research.

One evening, we were chatting in the hospital's small—and currently empty—emergency room when a thin, older woman strode through the creaking double doors. Wringing her hands, she told Dr. Edwin that her daughter, Irene, had been laboring in the birthing room for hours and was in great pain. "I want to take her to La Paz to get a C-section," she insisted.

"Why?" asked Dr. Edwin. "We can attend to her here, together with the partera."

"Aquí no hay atención," she muttered. "Here, there is no care."

"How can you say that when I'm right here?" The doctor smiled, but I sensed a tension in his voice. "I will go see how she is doing," he reassured the woman. "If you really want, we can send her to La Paz to get a C-section. But I think she is almost ready to give birth."

He told her to wait for him in the birthing room, but she continued to hover anxiously outside the double doors as he packed away his papers. "People have changed," he grumbled to me. "Before, women were afraid to have surgery, because they worried it would affect their ability to work on the farm. Now, they are asking for C-sections."[4]

The mother and I followed Dr. Edwin as he strode down the narrow hallway to the culturally adapted birthing room. Inside, Irene, the young woman giving birth, was kneeling on the floor, wrapped in a blanket, resting her forehead against the bed frame. Julia, one of the parteras working in the hospital, knelt on the wooden boards next to her. She rubbed Irene's lower back in a slow, firm motion, then motioned for Irene's husband, Ernesto, to do the same. Hesitantly, he imitated her movements, rubbing through the thick blanket as Irene continued to cry out in pain from her contractions. Julia explained to Ernesto that massaging would help ease the pain and move the baby downward.

While the three of them knelt on the floor by the bed, Irene's mother joined two other young women—Irene's sisters—who were sitting on the second bed amid a pile of blankets, baby clothes, snacks, and other items they had brought from home. Dr. Edwin turned to them and asked them to wait outside. Only one family member, the husband, could stay. As they reluctantly left the room, the doctor asked Julia and Ernesto to help Irene back onto the bed so that he could examine her.

They clumsily helped her to her feet and rolled her back onto the long black tarp stretched across the length of the bed. When she was in position, Dr. Edwin sat on the edge of the bed to examine her. It would not be much longer, he told her. Maybe another thirty minutes.

The doctor continued to perch on the edge of the bed, waiting for some movement. He turned to me and began telling me about the Master's in Public Health program he had done in Spain. Occasionally, he interrupted his narrative to place his hand on Irene's stomach and time her contractions on his Nokia flip phone. Julia had momentarily left the room to take a call, but Ernesto sat on the pillow next to his wife, cradling her forehead and whispering quietly to her. Dr. Edwin asked him teasingly how he had met his wife and whether he treated her well. Embarrassed, Ernesto looked down and murmured that they had met in high school.

The nurse and intern came in rolling a tray of medical supplies, and Dr. Edwin stood up to don a green mask and gown, much like Dr. Verónica had. Julia, meanwhile, returned and put on a deep orange gown that had been a gift from GHA to the hospital parteras.

Julia held Irene's hand and murmured to her, while Dr. Edwin went to the foot of the bed and told Irene to push. After several painful attempts, he asked her, "Would you rather give birth squatting? Sometimes it's easier that way."

Irene shook her head faintly. She continued to push, and at long last the baby began emerging. Dr. Edwin carefully pulled the newborn boy out and handed him to the intern, who placed him on the corner of the bed to rub him down and give him eye droplets. As Dr. Edwin then began to remove the placenta, he asked the couple whether they wanted to keep it. They both nodded. Turning to me, he explained, "You see, these are the customs of this place. They bury the placenta in a corner of the house after birth."

He was not yet done working when the other family members, who had been waiting outside the door, came into the room. Irene's mother-in-law carried a large pot of soup, which she placed on the gas burner in the corner. While I rarely saw the kitchenette in use (as the plates and dishes had also been locked away in the cabinet), some, like Irene's family, brought their own supplies and sought to use it to prepare the kinds of soups women needed to consume after birth. Irene's sister, meanwhile, picked up the bundled newborn and began cooing over him. Irritated by the commotion, Dr. Edwin asked them to wait outside until he was finished and to leave the baby with his mother.

For Dr. Edwin and others, the imitation of home-birthing practices made possible a different kind of care—one that was gentler and more reflective of patient desires. Cristiana Giordano (2014) argues that cultural recognition, even as it fixes and reifies, also operates as a therapeutic tool, facilitating new social relationships with patients. Doctors sought to make their patients feel well during birth—imagining this well-being primarily in terms of narratives about patients' alienation from the institutions of modernity.

Yet warm care also had a varied relationship to biomedical expertise. On the one hand, it facilitated biomedical work by ostensibly bringing patients into the hospital and making them feel more comfortable in the doctor's presence. On the other, practitioners still sought to circumscribe cultural difference when they perceived it to interfere with their ability to intervene effectively. Dr. Edwin might allow the husband to stay, but he quickly grew frustrated when other family members came in before he was finished. Cultural adaptation was thus linked to other practices in the hospital through their shared assumptions about the need to make culture manageable to save lives. Warmth operated as an affective strategy for practitioners to both address and mitigate patient desires in the hospital.

Like the GHA staffers, Dr. Edwin situated patient well-being within a bounded notion of culture. He approached his work with a checklist of questions, informed by his cultural sensitivity training. Did Irene want to give birth with the help of a midwife? Did she want to give birth squatting? Did she want to take the placenta home? These were questions, as Dr. Edwin put it, that sought to address "the customs of this place." Rather than silencing patient desires, he wanted to give voice to them—so long as they fit within his notions of what constituted cultural authenticity. He grumbled that women were not like they once were; now, they wanted cesareans instead of birth with a midwife. He was particularly taken aback when Irene's mother declared, despite his offers, that "here, there is no care." By providing this kind of choice filled with expectation, he sought to engage patients' practices in terms that were legible to him as a practitioner, with little room for uncertainty or incommensurability.

The asking of questions was also closely tied to material and bodily practices, as doctors sought to mimic certain elements of the home. Take the wooden bed, juxtaposed to the gurney in the other room. On the bed, Dr. Edwin explained proudly, the warmer, softer blankets would make women feel more comfortable, and they could give birth in various positions. His own positioning changed as well. Rather than standing at a distance while waiting out the contractions, he sat on the corner of the bed alongside Irene. Even as he intervened as a doctor (timing the contractions, delivering the baby, and cutting the cord), he combined this with what he described as warmer practices. Yet his efforts to create intimacy—by asking Irene questions of how she wanted to give birth, or teasing Ernesto about his marriage—were met with hesitation.

Allowing room for other kinds of care, for psychological support, was essential to saving lives, Dr. Edwin argued. It was the only means to convince women to come to the hospital. He showed me a graph of data he had collected over the years: two increasing lines demonstrating, he explained, that ever since the culturally adapted rooms were constructed, more women were coming to the hospital to give birth. His reliance on apoyo psicológico ultimately extended—rather than disrupted—the ingrained logics of rural biomedicine by working to bring Indigenous women into the clinical space.

THE LABOR OF WARM CARE

As biomedical practitioners drew boundaries around how warmth could enter the hospital, they also delegated much of the work of apoyo psicológico to parteras assisting with births. At the time of my research, three Aymara parteras—Julia, Lucinda, and Tomasa—worked in the hospital. While they continued caring for pregnant women outside the hospital and assisting in home births, they also showed up for regularly scheduled shifts in the hospital. However, they, along with their traditional healer colleagues (see Chapter 4), did not receive salaries for their work in the institution. They continued nonetheless to show up for shifts because hospital affiliation offered them new forms of legitimacy, particularly in a context in which they continued to face marginalization and discrimination; many also hoped that hospital affiliation might eventually translate into other resources, support, and forms of social mobility. Yet as they were brought as unwaged labor into the hospital, parteras were primarily expected to take on feminized psychological support work that might sustain—but not replace—biomedical obstetric interventions.

In this final section, I examine how parteras' relational, temperature-based practices were rerouted and absorbed as uncompensated, racialized and gendered labor necessary to maintaining the hospital's warm care. These forms of labor denied the role of parteras as experts who could intervene in difficult births, instead positioning them as undertaking secondary affective and psychological support work that would sustain biomedical intervention. Simultaneously, the reliance on apoyo psicológico from parteras to maintain warm care negated the role of husbands and other family members. Nonetheless, parteras as well as family members were able to engage some elements of warm care to craft moments of intimacy and partially reaffirm the material and relational care of the home.

After the Alma Ata Accords in 1978, global health and development programs increasingly encouraged health institutions in the Global South to work with "traditional birth attendants"—local birth practitioners who gained their knowledge primarily through experiential and community-based routes—with the idea that they might also be trained in some basic biomedical techniques and refer patients with complications to biomedical institutions (Dixon 2020; El Kotni 2019; Guerra-Reyes 2019; Vega 2018). Yet such policies often glossed over the complexity of local birthing practices (Pinto 2008).[5] Within the past few decades, moreover, global policy initiatives have also created new divisions that privileged midwives who have been institutionally trained (often called "skilled birth attendants"). These programs have often excluded parteras who gained their knowledge from community sources (Dixon 2020; El Kotni 2019; Guerra-Reyes 2019) or have seen them as valuable primarily because of the caring dimensions of their practice, rather than their expertise (Pinto 2008). These divisions, moreover, have failed to account for the ways that many contemporary midwives blur these lines and obtained knowledge from multiple sources (Dixon 2020).[6]

In Bolivia, where programs to recruit and train Indigenous parteras had been in place since the 1970s (Gallien 2015; Kimball 2020), similar dynamics unfolded. Yet some key differences also existed between Bolivian health policies under Morales and other moves toward intercultural birthing elsewhere in the region. In contrast to some other countries (Guerra-Reyes 2019), for example, Bolivian health policies allowed home births, even if they encouraged women to give birth in clinical settings. Therefore, parteras could continue to provide care in patients' homes rather than being obliged to work exclusively in institutional settings. Although officials placed a heavy emphasis on credentialing nonbiomedical practitioners and rendering them legible to the state, they also insisted on the importance of recognizing multiple kinds of medical knowledge and practice.

Alongside this flexibility, however, intercultural birthing, when put into practice, also involved transforming parteras into (mostly uncompensated) care workers who could sustain the warmth of the hospital. On the Bolivian Altiplano, as I have detailed, experienced community members had long lent their expertise in the process of childbirth. Many of these same individuals were identified and trained by development organizations in ways that demarcated them as parteras for policy. Julia described to me how she began to learn how to care for women during childbirth by watching her father help her mother during the birth of her younger siblings. Later, after successfully helping her own sister give birth, Julia had begun developing a reputation in her village as someone who was skilled in assisting births. She was called upon to help with several other births in her village before she was recruited by an NGO for training that taught her how to identify risk factors for complications during birth, before eventually being recruited to work in the hospital. Others related similar stories: they already had been aiding in birth in their communities, they were invited to participate in NGO or state workshops, and they increasingly began working in collaboration with local clinics and hospitals.

These recruitment efforts drew rigid boundaries around who was assumed to be a partera and what kinds of work they did. State and NGO categorizations often left out husbands as well as yatiris who did not fit within the institutional expectation of the partera. These gendered categorizations also had implications for parteras who were recruited. Several parteras engaged in other healing practices including and beyond care related to reproduction—yet institutions slotted them into a more narrowly defined role of assisting births.[7] Lucinda, for example, also practiced as a *naturista* (natural healer), but was only on the books as a partera in the hospital. As I continue to elaborate in the next chapter, both male traditional healers and female parteras provided uncompensated labor for the hospital—yet they faced different institutional expectations of the kinds of labor they should be performing. More so than their male colleagues, parteras were expected to provide psychological support and do the work of warm care for their patients. Parteras' assistive role might include care practices such as soothing patients, engaging in cultural and linguistic translation, and making patients feel included.

Institutional expectations around psychological support reflected gendered and racialized assumptions about who undertook care work and how. Biomedical physicians working in the Machacamarca Hospital sometimes made assessments about parteras' affective dispositions, remarking on which ones were *dulce* ("sweet") and which ones were more combative and *renegonas* ("complainers"), thus more difficult to work with. Such commentaries reflected not only perceptions of affect and disposition, but were also connected to language, as physicians often deemed parteras who primarily spoke Aymara and did not speak Spanish to be more difficult. Scholars working in a range of contexts have noted that the feminization and racialization of labor often entail ascribing specific attributes, dispositions, and embodied signs to groups of workers (Chatterjee 2001; Salzinger 2003; Ong 2010). As Sareeta Amrute argues, this process of ascribing characteristics also means that racialized subjects "are bulked together as a group of workers who are able because of their cultural capacities to do [this kind of work]" (2016, 2). In qualifying the affective dispositions of parteras, biomedical practitioners evaluated partera labor primarily in terms of their gendered and racialized affective capacity to be "warm" with patients.

As with other forms of warm care in the Machacamarca Hospital, hospital administrators and biomedical practitioners also drew boundaries around what kinds of work parteras could and could not undertake in the hospital. Echoing the engagements with warmth I have described in this chapter, biomedical practitioners positioned parteras as potential sources of risk to patients who might be allowed in on limited terms. Under Bolivian intercultural health policy, patients were in principle able to choose whether they wanted a biomedical doctor or a partera to deliver their child. Many hospital practitioners, however, expressed concerns about the legal and health risks posed by giving too much leeway to parteras. As Dr. Verónica told me, "The law is now such that responsibility [if something goes wrong] falls on the doctor. There's no law that the partera gets sanctioned if something goes wrong. There is nothing. So, I can't risk so much working with the partera." In turn, others, like Dr. Edwin, who were more open to collaborations, emphasized parteras' value in helping patients feel comfortable and supported. However, they continued to insist that while parteras could be present in an assistive capacity, the biomedical doctor was the one who needed to deliver the infant.

The affective dimensions of recognition—articulated in the Machacamarca Hospital in terms of warm rooms and the promise of a new, more inclusive care—thus also relied on the uneven distribution of care labor within ongoing capitalist projects. Marxist feminist scholars have long drawn attention to women's household labor as a key site of social reproduction—that is, of societal continuity and well-being. Domestic care practices (including, for example, childbirth and childrearing) sustain the reproduction of labor power and capitalist systems more broadly, yet also go undervalued and uncompensated.[8] While socially reproductive labor can also take many forms beyond women's domestic work, it is also no coincidence that both women and the domestic space of the home were being associated in this case with supplementary forms of care that did not require compensation. The expectation that parteras take on gendered affective labor extended entrenched devaluations of women's work in the home.

At the same time, parteras' care practices were never fully subsumed into dominant biomedical systems. While biomedical providers frequently interpreted parteras' care practices as psychological support work, these practices also emerged from parteras' expertise in childbirth. Together, parteras, patients, and their husbands were also able to create small moments of relationality during childbirth that could both align with and subvert dominant expectations of warm care.

One afternoon in the culturally adapted birthing room, a young woman named Elena was enduring painful contractions. While the biomedical doctor was out of the room—he stepped in only occasionally to time the contractions—one of the hospital parteras, Lucinda, helped Elena off the bed and onto the floor. An elderly Aymara woman, Lucinda had learned how to care for women in pregnancy and childbirth from her grandmother, but later attended several state and NGO workshops designed to train traditional birth attendants in basic biomedical techniques. Now, she gestured at Elena to lean her forehead against the side of the wooden bed. Kneeling behind Elena, her long layered skirts pooled around her, Lucinda moved her knotted hands in a slow, circular motion over Elena's lower back to ease the pain of her contractions, much as Julia had done for Irene.

For biomedical practitioners, parteras' lower-back massages were a form of soothing that was relatively harmless; it would not interfere with obstetric intervention, and moreover, it seemed to calm patients, especially as they were waiting out contractions. (They were less certain about parteras' other methods, and rarely allowed them to be practiced in the hospital—for example, arguing that manteo could injure the fetus, or that the administration of teas could cause complications). But for parteras and patients, bodily care techniques such as massages were not simply a means to soothe patients or quell fears; rather, they became a means to facilitate a good birth and also draw others into relation. As Elena continued to endure her contractions, for example, Lucinda called over Elena's husband and showed him how he could give massages as well. Such care practices placed intimate, embodied relations at the heart of childbirth in ways that exceeded a narrow racialized and gendered definition of psychological support.

Thus, even amid these institutional constraints, warmth took on multiple forms for patients, shifting between commensurability and incommensurability with hospital procedures. Husbands, although not allowed to take on a more central role, sat on the edge of the bed and held their wives' foreheads. Midwives gave patients massages on their lower back to ease the pain of contractions. Extended family members brought a pot of soup to put on the stove after birth. Warm air, materials, and touch helped create vital intimacy and ease pain— even as they could not always fully maintain bodily wellness, or fully transform the conditions of obstetric violence in the hospital.

In this context, parteras also leveraged their positions to legitimate their practice and assert their expertise. While many expressed frustrations with their ongoing marginalization within formal systems of health care delivery, they also saw intercultural policies as an important step forward to being taken seriously. In one memorable moment (the only time I encountered something of the sort), I came across Lucinda teaching a young biomedical intern how to massage a patient. The intern, in her early twenties, had recently completed her medical training and was on the obligatory three-month rotation to a rural health establishment required to receive a medical degree in Bolivia. While patients were waiting out contractions, interns were often left to watch over the patient and call one of the staff physicians if something went awry. Most of the time, they sat quietly in the corner looking at their phones, occasionally getting up to check on the patient. Lucinda, however, asked the intern that day if she wanted to learn how to give massages. The intern shyly nodded, and the two women crouched on either side of the patient kneeling against the bed, Lucinda showing her how to massage the patient's lower back through the thick blanket.

In her powerful critique of development experts who purport to offer "cultural adaptation" as a solution to inequalities in maternal health in Latin America, Beatriz Loza argues that approaching cultural adaptation as a simple technical fix is insufficient. As she writes, "In Bolivia, for example, there have been experiments in [cultural adaptation] with few encouraging results; for if hospitals have been transformed in their decorations, the quality of care continues to be undesirable" (2013, 1085, my translation). I am largely in agreement with her argument about the continuities of obstetric violence and inadequate care under conditions of cultural adaptation. Yet rather than approaching cultural adaptation as a superficial decoration—a mere shell—we might turn our attention to how these continuities were intentionally built, made to allow new forms of warmth, but only insofar as they maintained the functioning of the hospital as such. Architecturally distinct spaces were made to reinscribe the rural hospital as a space for managing Indigenous life.

When I asked women about their experiences using the culturally adapted room, the most common response—echoing like a worn refrain—was that it was *bien no más* ("just okay"). This response differed from the more triumphalist accounts of Bolivian intercultural birthing that appeared in international news coverage and transnational aid circuits, which often centered representations of newly grateful and self-actualized Aymara patients. Instead, "bien no más" was a kind of verbal shrug; it carried resonances with the invocations of "not good enough" that Simpson (2020, 5) describes in response to settler offers of sympathy and repair. It was a reminder that if warmth was central to well-being, in its current institutional form, it maintained continuities with the spaces and practices of violent intervention in the hospital.

Warmth could be appealing, preferable to purely cold interventions; the culturally adapted rooms in the Machacamarca Hospital could at times be sites of intimacy and rest. As I have shown, patients did sometimes seek out and engage meaningfully with aspects of the warm birthing room: a patient's husband saw it as a space where he was allowed to be present; another patient's mother-in-law sought to use the stove to heat soups central to healing the body after birth. Parteras found new ways to assert their expertise and sustain patient well-being, even as they were constrained in their roles. At the same time, ethnographic attention to the rooms suggests that there is more slippage between warm and cold than one might initially assume. Warm temperatures—able during labor to offer bodily comfort and ease pain—also facilitated ongoing forms of harsh biomedical care during birth.

In this chapter, I have examined how warm hospital architectures enabled and enacted racialized sensory, affective, and "psychological" care work. This is work that flattened and refigured the ways that temperature circulated in home birth, in ways that rendered it commensurate with and drew boundaries around what kind of care could enter the hospital. Practitioners couched measures—having patients lie on the bed, allowing a husband to be present, or simply absorbing the warm air—in terms of new kindness and inclusivity, of letting patients give birth "as they wanted." Yet many hospital practitioners were also concerned that allowing too much warmth into the hospital would disrupt their ability to intervene effectively in patient bodies. Warmth as psychological support was acceptable; warmth as a material force, less so.

Simultaneously, enacting these forms of warmth-as-psychological support also depended on the uncompensated, gendered and racialized labor of parteras. Institutions and providers expected parteras to embody warmth—to have a supportive disposition and to help quell patient fears during birth. But in slotting parteras into the role of psychological support, institutional actors erased their expertise, as well as the role of others involved in caregiving during childbirth, such as husbands and extended family members. Still, parteras as well as patients and family members also rerouted the conditions of the birthing room to their own ends; while practices in the hospital were not the same as in the home, they were often able to carve out small moments of intimacy and support.

4 EMBODIED REDISTRIBUTION

Extraction and the Labor of Healing

WHEN I WALKED WITH REYNALDO around the Machacamarca Municipal Hospital's medicinal plant greenhouse one day in mid-2015, he was worried. An older Aymara man, convert to Evangelical Protestantism, and *naturista* (natural healer or naturopath), Reynaldo had been working in the highland Bolivian hospital for nearly a decade. GHA had built the greenhouse in the early 2000s with the idea that healers could grow and harvest plants for medicinal purposes. Yet as we talked, Reynaldo gazed in frustration at the rows of medicinal plants. The rue, chamomile, hierba buena, and other plants sprouting from the beds were worn and droopy. Small white insects buzzed in clouds around some of the bushes. He wondered out loud whether biomedical practitioners working in the hospital ripped leaves off the plants for their own use.

As we continued the conversation, it became clear that the decimated plants were part of a broader host of frustrations about the mismatch between state promises of decolonized health care and their implementation on the ground. Reynaldo described problems wrought by lack of material support for the four traditional healers working in the hospital, noting that the exam room that had been designated for them was also threadbare.[1] Most important, healers did not receive a salary for their work in the hospital; unlike their biomedical colleagues, they did not receive any formal compensation from the institution. Hearing his litany of concerns helped me to revisit his earlier speculations that perhaps his biomedical colleagues had been ripping leaves off the medicinal plants for their own use. No one had seen biomedical doctors doing it, but for Reynaldo and other healers, it might be happening, it might explain the state of the plants. As I came to better understand over the course of this and other conversations with healers, decimated medicinal plants were not only a marker of unequal dynamics between paid and unpaid medical laborers in the hospital. They also pointed to anxieties about a lack of material sustenance and relations required to nourish patient well-being.

This chapter examines how healers grappling with conditions of exploitation sought to pull Bolivian state, medical, and nonprofit institutions into anticipatory relations that I call *embodied redistribution*. When healing patients, they situated institutions alongside other human and more-than-human relations that could either sustain or impede patient well-being; they vocally demanded that the state materially invest in salaries, supplies, and maintenance to nourish relations essential to healing. Through these hopeful practices of embodied redistribution, healers redefined state promises of material redistribution as a moral obligation to care for embodied relations and counter the illness-inducing effects of alienation. In healers' framing, material redistribution would facilitate healing relations between patients and both human and other-than-human beings. In turn, they construed state failure to act on these obligations as processes of extraction at the root of many illnesses.

The appropriation of healer labor paralleled the uncompensated labor of parteras that I described in Chapter 3, although they unfolded differently along lines of gender. A majority of professionalized healers I interviewed (both in and out of the hospital context) were men, although I interviewed several healers who were women as well. Among practitioners I interviewed working in the hospital, Lucinda, the partera who figured into Chapter 3, was also trained as a naturista; she co-ran a private consultorio with her husband, Reynaldo, and also regularly dispensed medical advice to patients. However, in the hospital she was only on the books as a partera. Both men and women practiced healing (Loza 2008), and in some forms of ritual healing, men and women were also understood to have different healing powers and roles (Burman 2017). But with the professionalization and institutionalization of healing practice since the 1980s, men were also taking on more visible leadership roles within the healer unions that advocated for healing practice. These dynamics exceeded state and NGO recruitment of healers but were often replicated in hospital and clinical settings.

I suggest that practices of embodied redistribution reflected shifting concerns in the rural but urbanizing town of Machacamarca around the bodily effects of commodification and alienation from relations, as well as who was responsible for restoring well-being. Like a growing number of nonbiomedical practitioners around the world, Indigenous healers from a range of specialties in Bolivia had been increasingly pursuing avenues of training, professionalization, and certification to legitimate their practice, particularly since the formal legalization of their status in the 1980s.[2] Yet for at least some patients, the commodification and professionalization of healing had also made it less efficacious—as they understood healers to be increasingly divorced from the human and other-than-human relations that had long been at the core of their practice. State officials, too, picked up this narrative, albeit on different terms: even as new laws increasingly required healers to adopt norms of professionalization, officials often positioned more authentic forms of healing as those that operated outside the market economy. In keeping with this framing, some officials also suggested that healers' demands for compensation were spurious because they did not reflect the perspectives of all healers. I show how professionalized healers, in contrast, resituated as yet unfulfilled state investments as essential to sustaining the human and more-than-human relations at the core of their practice. In short, they argued that their lack of efficacy was not a shortcoming in their own practice, but a result of enduring extractions from institutions.

I argue that as healers sought to bring institutions into embodied relations, they sought to link questions of cultural recognition with those of redistribution, even as they reformulated them in new ways. Globally, scholars have heavily debated whether cultural recognition or material redistribution offers a more substantial path to transformation (Fraser and Honneth 2003)—even though, as Yellowknives Dene political theorist Glenn Coulthard (2014) suggests, the very terms of this debate largely solidify the settler state as the primary vehicle of justice, negating possibilities that Indigenous nations might determine their own paths to transformation.[3] In Bolivia, resonant debates have for decades taken shape between Marxist critics of capitalism and class inequality on the one hand (Zavaleta Mercado 2018) and Indianist calls to attend to Indigenous worlds and the effects of enduring colonialism on the other (Reinaga 1969). Yet while these perspectives have sometimes been in friction with one another, numerous activist projects have also sought to place these approaches in conversation with one another, acknowledging how historically rooted dynamics of land dispossession and labor exploitation have often gone hand in hand in Bolivia. These projects have ranged, for example, from Katarista movement efforts in the 1970s to link class and ethnic struggle (Sanjinés 2004) to efforts in the 1990s and early 2000s by the intellectual collective Grupo Comuna to bridge Marxist and Indianist approaches (García Linera, Gutierrez, Prada, and Tapia 1999). These efforts were also influential for the Morales administration, which sought to combine a deepening of Indigenous cultural and territorial autonomy with state-led redistribution of resources (Postero 2007; 2017; Maclean 2023). Yet when implemented in state policy, both of these projects encountered limitations, as MAS officials heavily circumscribed the terms of cultural recognition and as state redistributive projects remained constrained by limited funding and fragmentary infrastructures. Especially when it came to the inclusion of healers and parteras in the health care system, state officials often positioned a narrow and reified cultural recognition of healing relations as a way to deflect from questions of monetary compensation. They positioned warm care and inclusion of healers as compensation enough.

In this chapter, I trace how healers confronted these limitations by positioning ontologies of healing in and of themselves as a central ground on which to make claims for state redistribution. That is, rather than pitting recognition of Indigenous healing practices against questions of monetary compensation, they suggested that the state (and adjacent medical and nonprofit institutions) had a wider moral obligation to care for the relations that facilitated healing. In doing so, they largely retained intact state authority to enact transformation, but sought to hold that authority more accountable to relations and reroute it into forms that were more livable in the context of Machacamarca. As Métis anthropologist Zoe Todd (2018) suggests, encounters with the state often require negotiating the state's political and legal ideologies, but Indigenous nations also rework, diffuse, and refract these ideologies through local relations with human and other-than-human beings. Healers engaged—but ultimately challenged—state officials' capacity to determine the scope of well-being by asserting the conditions they would need to care for others effectively.

COMMODIFICATION, REDISTRIBUTION, AND THE SOURCES OF INEFFICACY

Nonbiomedical practices of healing had long been a mainstay of care in rural Aymara and Quechua villages in the Bolivian Andes, often integrated into local systems of gifting and exchange (Crandon-Malamud 1991). Yet ways of approaching health had been changing rapidly for both healers and their patients through multiple waves of rural-to-urban migration that also increasingly brought people into a capitalist market economy. Healing practices became increasingly commodified—and also became a central, if contested, ground for grappling with the bodily effects of wider political-economic transitions.

After the National Revolution of 1952, the Bolivian government formally abolished the hacienda system that Spanish colonizers and their descendants had set up to control land and conscript labor in the areas around Machacamarca, as elsewhere in the Bolivian Andes (Dunkerley 1984). Yet state redistribution of land to Indigenous campesinos, while a significant step toward reparation, did not always lead to conditions for thriving; land parcels were small and fragmented, and a severe drought made making a living from agriculture difficult. Aymara and Quechua campesinos, now free to buy and sell their labor power, started moving to urban centers to find work (Albó, Sandoval, and Greaves 1981). Another wave of rural-to-urban migration—that also drove people to smaller regional towns like Machacamarca—took shape in the 1980s when neoliberal structural adjustment measures flexibilized labor, closed many mines, and left miners unemployed (Kohl and Farthing 2006; Gill 2000; Lazar 2008). At the time of my research, the town of Machacamarca had about eleven thousand residents and had been undergoing a process of rural urbanization for several decades. Most residents worked in the informal economy, selling goods at local markets or driving transport, although many still continued to maintain plots of land in their home villages.

Many newly arrived residents of Machacamarca sought socioeconomic mobility via the accumulation of wealth and participation in an urban informal market economy. In Bolivia, as I described in Chapter 2, racialized and classed mobility were often linked, as access to education, professionalization, and salaried labor were also tied to social whitening. Yet these long-standing configurations were also being partially subverted with the rise of a new Aymara middle and upper class, particularly in larger cities like El Alto. Some networks of Aymara traders had become prosperous through their trade in second-hand and contraband goods, including electronics, household appliances, cellphones, and clothing (Tassi 2010; 2017). Although Machacamarca was a much smaller center—and still closely connected to rural farmlands—many residents of the town likewise actively sought to enter informal trade networks in the hopes of gaining socioeconomic stability and greater access to goods. Moreover, for many residents of Machacamarca, the potential for growing prosperity was also helped along by the Morales administration's social investments and redistributive projects. New state investments in conditional cash transfers, combined with often highly publicized ceremonies inaugurating new public infrastructures, raised hopes among many in Machacamarca that the Morales administration was moving away from a politics of state abandonment and was willing to sustain people's economic well-being.

Yet even as new possibilities for mobility were opening up, many Aymara residents were nonetheless left behind in Bolivia's economic boom. As Susan Ellison argues, individuals still reckoned with enduring discrimination and challenges to obtaining mobility as the "racial partitioning that enables capitalist extraction" (2023, 5) persisted. And the state's redistributive program, while it had significant impacts, also encountered limitations of funding and fragmentary infrastructure. In Machacamarca, many of my neighbors described how they had shed the deep poverty of their rural childhoods, yet making ends meet could often still be difficult. Some held Evo Morales directly responsible for improvements in their circumstances—but also, in turn, pointed to his shortcomings when state support was not always enough to mitigate ongoing economic vicissitudes. My neighbor Rosa, a MAS voter, was anxious that a rapid drop in quinoa prices in 2015 had made it harder for her family to earn a steady income from regional market sales; the hardship caused by a drop in prices, she worried, also meant that many people *ya no lo quieren al Evo* ("don't love Evo anymore"). Yet years later, in 2022, when I went back to visit her, Rosa had a different story to tell: newly elected President Arce (who, like Evo Morales, represented the MAS), was a decent president, but not as good as Evo. When Evo was around, the municipalities had more money (*había plata*); now, the funds had dried up. For her and many others I interviewed, the state carried partial responsibility for the flows of money that might sustain well-being.

Scholars have pointed out how Aymara migrants to urban areas operated neither fully inside nor fully outside of capitalism and instead brought together plural systems of value and exchange (Maclean 2023; Tassi 2017; Yampara et al. 2007). For example, traders often engaged in active free-market competition and accumulation of wealth, yet they also combined these with conspicuous displays of abundance, generosity, and redistribution—such as investing in communal fiestas—that were understood to have both economic and relational significance (Tassi 2010; 2017). Likewise, rural-to-urban migrants engaged in market-based practices but also hoped that the state might sustain them through redistributive projects—an expectation that reflected long-standing practices of patronage and exchange across social hierarchies. These practices, while sometimes subject to disagreement and contestation,[4] often centered the idea that those with more resources or power should engage in morally appropriate forms of redistribution (Winchell 2022). If capitalism itself is rarely totalizing and depends on "unstable, contingent networks" (Bear, Ho, Tsing, and Yanagisako 2015),[5] residents of Machacamarca were continually and creatively reworking economic forms. Yet as I show in the following pages, engaging with these different forms could also have effects for healing and the body itself.

Healers followed trajectories similar to that of many other recent migrants to the town of Machacamarca, adapting elements of their practice to an urbanizing market economy. Many opened private *consultorios* (offices, exam rooms) and began selling medicinal plant concoctions to make ends meet. Particularly after the legal recognition of their practice in 1984, many also began pursuing opportunities for formal training, certification, and professionalization. Yet processes of commodification could create opportunities while also raising new preoccupations.

Historically, healing practices had derived their efficacy from cultivating reciprocal and redistributive relations among human and other-than-human beings. In this context, relations of exchange were understood to be at once ethical, material, and ontological. More broadly, widespread practices of exchanging food, money, and labor were understood to constitute moral personhood (Canessa 2012) and also materially sustain a well body. As Marisol de la Cadena (2015) has argued in her work in the Peruvian Andes, ontologies are actively constituted through relations; that is, entities (such as earth beings, persons, and in this case, the body itself) come into being through the relations that enact them.[6] Healers, especially in more rural areas, had often been tasked with cultivating relations with both human and other-than-human beings to ensure corporeal well-being—for example, by regularly making offerings to sentient earth beings that inhabited the landscape, or by treating ailments caused by envy (Tapias 2015) or other ruptures in social relations (Canessa 2012). Shifting into a more commodified market economy—in which healers bought and sold their services as well as medicinal plant remedies—could sometimes provoke anxieties among both healers and their patients that healing was becoming too deracinated from the relations that made it effective. If bodies were understood to be intimately co-constituted through relations with human and other-than-human entities, dominant liberal capitalist and colonial models often relied on the separation of beings into decontextualized, autonomous subjects (Goeman 2015; Lara 2020; Yazzie 2018).[7]

Even so, as Mei Zhan has argued, while processes of commodification and rationalization can transform traditional medical practice, they rarely entail a complete erasure of past practices; instead, traditional medical practitioners navigating new market economies "negotiate new forms of knowledge and redefine areas of expertise" (2009, 72). Aymara healers especially emphasized the value of professionalizing and commodifying their practice, which they tied not only to facilitating socioeconomic mobility, but also enabling their practice to finally be legitimated on equal footing with biomedical practitioners' knowledge. Commodification, for them, could often be a way to rearticulate the value of healing in new forms. At the same time, they also sought to highlight enduring continuities with the forms of healing they had undertaken in more rural settings (Loza 2008; Sikkink 2010) and emphasized how their practice might also help address new ills emerging with the process of urbanization. Yet questions of how to engage commodification—and how to reassert forms of life-making—were also highly contested, as healers from different specialties articulated different ontologies of healing and relation to the surrounding landscape.

Patricio, an older Aymara man and sole ritual healer to work in the Machacamarca Hospital, was originally from a small village in the province of Inquisivi. He gained his healing abilities after surviving a lightning strike and practiced for many years as a *yatiri* (Aymara for "one who knows"). He healed the sick, divined the future, and cultivated relations with earth beings and ancestral spirits.[8] He was a Catholic, although, like many people living in the Andes, he combined this practice comfortably with his enduring relations with a sentient landscape (Orta 2004). After he moved to Machacamarca, he continued to treat patients for problems like fright and soul loss. But he also started to sell teas and pomades based in medicinal plants. He had already worked with plants back in his home village—but learned new techniques for packaging them and selling them when taking a traditional medicine certification course in the city of La Paz under the auspices of the Bolivian Society for Traditional and Ancestral Medicine (SOBOMETRA), an organization that had been formalized with the legalization of traditional medical practice in 1984. Still, he worried sometimes that his neighbors were forgetting relations that had long been central to their healing and well-being.[9] They no longer sought to "reach the Pachamama," Patricio explained, naming an important earth being responsible for the well-being of both bodies and lands. Notably, a number of ritual healers I interviewed refused to participate in the process of commodification and professionalization entirely, suggesting that doing so ran contrary to the ways they were accustomed to practicing healing. My acquaintance Incarna was an elderly ritual healer who lived in a village about a twenty-minute drive from Machacamarca. She did not work in the hospital, nor did she seek out any kind of formal credentialing. Instead, she continued to occasionally see people who sought her help in her home; in the village, she had a reputation as someone who was knowledgeable, who could read coca, who could call back souls. In contrast to Incarna, Patricio actively embraced entry into a system of capitalist exchange, but often continued to express tension and ambivalence about the effects on his healing.

Patricio's three naturista colleagues in the hospital, however, had a different perspective. *Naturismo* (natural healing or naturopathy) was an emergent healing practice that had grown in popularity especially in urban and recently urbanizing areas like Machacamarca. Many naturistas were Aymara rural-to-urban migrants who had converted to Evangelical Protestantism, a fast-growing religion that preached against the existence of sentient earth beings (see Van Vleet 2011). Naturistas were not faith healers, but they frequently drew on Evangelical tenets that tied clean and healthy living to the moral good (Hardin 2018). They pulled together elements of Andean Indigenous herbal medicine, Chinese herbalism, New Age spirituality, and other nonbiomedical therapies in the preparation and sale of teas, pomades, steam baths, and massages (Sikkink 2010). They also often positioned themselves as treating many of the same ailments that biomedicine did, especially chronic and metabolic ailments that they described as increasing with urban living.

In their recounting, land was not sentient—but rupture from land-based living was nonetheless a key source of illness in urban areas: as people were increasingly exposed to chemicals and toxins, as they ate junk foods and foods without a clear origin, and as they no longer lived from the land, they were getting sicker. For many naturistas, com-modified medicinal plant remedies could in themselves help patients reestablish ties with a more natural, landed past. In many ways, their practice paralleled the growing global popularity of market-based herbals, which, as Stacey Langwick (2018) has suggested, reflect ef-forts to create more "habitable worlds" amid growing concerns with economic precarity and toxicity. Segundo, an older Aymara man and an Evangelical pastor, had worked as a biomedical nurse before later in life deciding to become a naturista. He explained how he had learned to use medicinal plants from his family, but much like Patricio had decided to take extra training and certification courses in the city to hone his knowledge. As Segundo explained, medicinal plants were just as efficacious as biomedical pharmaceuticals: "Our plants are also antibiotics. They are also anti-inflammatories." Yet, as he went on to qualify, they also worked more "slowly" and "gently" on the body. In contrast to Patricio, who identified more of a tension between heal-ing relations and commodification, Segundo positioned the medicinal plant commodity as condensing the very relations that made healing efficacious. These commodities worked more "gently" through their ostensible links to Indigenous land-based relations, in contrast to the harsh chemicals of pharmaceuticals that could also damage the body.

Many of my neighbors drew on multiple healing systems, including ritual healing, naturismo, and biomedicine. Echoing Libbet Crandon-Malamud's (1991) foundational study of medical pluralism in the Andes, people often combined and recombined therapies as a way to position themselves and forge social relationships. For Crandon-Malamud, forging social relationships through therapeutic choices also, in many instances, had extra-medical benefits of "gain[ing] access to resources, including both material goods and power" (31). Yet while questions of social mobility and access to resources were likewise key for my interlocutors, I also suggest that focusing narrowly on these aspects can neglect the often contradictory ways that people navigate shifting economic circumstances and dynamics of commodification. It can also miss how questions of resources are not simply extra-medical but might be understood to have embodied effects in and of themselves. Mareike Winchell (2018; 2022) has pointed out that studies of moral economy—including many studies of patronage in the Andes—often overemphasize relations as an instrumentalist quest for resources; in doing so, they can neglect how enduring practices of exchange entail deep-rooted ethical and affective attachments that can be flexibly recrafted across multiple sites. In Machacamarca, the question of access to resources was likewise not purely strategic, nor did it provide a rationally instrumentalist substrate to how people navigated healing (see Jašarević 2011; 2017).[10] The circulation of money and other resources could not be disentangled from people's moral expectations and how relations were also profoundly embodied.

These often contradictory moral expectations underpinned how residents of Machacamarca weighed the efficacy of healing practices. Many of my neighbors had shed the ritual relations with earth beings that had characterized their lives in rural villages, regardless of whether they had converted to Evangelical Protestantism. Even as they sought to retain many moral norms around exchange, they often described earth beings as entities that had characterized the lives of their parents and grandparents (thereby feeding into Patricio's concerns that many people were losing this particular mode of relation). As a result, healing methods like naturismo were also growing in popularity: naturistas positioned themselves as a more modern practice, even as they promised to help reestablish ties to a landed past. And yet, even as this modality of healing was growing in popularity, many of my neighbors worried that too much commodification of healing had made it less efficacious. They expressed skepticism of a practice that they viewed as too divorced from the relations essential to healing. Even for some Evangelical converts and people who no longer related to a sentient landscape, naturistas' commodification could make them less efficacious. Two of my neighbors, both Evangelical converts, criticized ritual healers of the past as "witches" (brujos) who engaged in superstitions. And yet, they noted, these very witches had at least been more efficacious. These days, they insisted, naturistas "were only interested in money."

Such hesitations and criticisms were not always limited to naturistas, however. Other neighbors described any healers affiliated with the hospital as carrileros—an idiomatic Bolivian Spanish word meaning "swindler" or "only concerned with money." Some of these town residents did not know that healers did not receive a salary—but positioned hospital affiliation as a sign that healers had broken with the very relations that made them efficacious.

These preoccupations that commodification had impeded the efficacy of healing had continuities with long-standing concerns with the ill effects of alienation and deracination. Even before Machacamarca had started growing in size and people had moved out of their more rural villages, ruptured relations were a key source of preoccupation and sickness. To this day, my neighbors explained, the site where a Spanish ore refining mill once stood on the river near Machacamarca remained haunted; strange fires burned at night and mysterious figures wandered about. One could go mad if one stumbled across the site accidentally. Scholars working with Indigenous communities in the Andes and elsewhere in Latin America have highlighted how the capitalist alienation from labor often manifests in the form of sickness-inducing devils and other monstrous creatures that haunt the landscape.[11] For Gastón Gordillo (2004), in conversation with Michael Taussig (2010), these dynamics show how Indigenous conceptions of fetishism also became a ground for theorizing commodity fetishism and the abstraction of social relations involved in capitalism. But these long-standing configurations, I suggest, also highlight how transitions—in lifeways and in bodies—could not always be easily mapped as a neatly linear progression from noncapitalist to capitalist relations, or from so-called "tradition" to "modernity" (see Palmié 2002; Latour 1993; Yates-Doerr 2015). Instead, ruptures in social relations had already been unfolding at multiple points in the past centuries, as Aymara villagers experienced layered forms of land dispossession and labor exploitation that deracinated them from relations. As people increasingly migrated to urban centers or participated in processes of rural urbanization, long-standing modes of interpreting illness often became a ground for interpreting new events (Tapias 2015).

These concerns about alienation of healing took shape even as many Machacamarqueños were themselves pursuing avenues of commodification and capitalist accumulation in the informal market economy. That is, most of my neighbors did not fully reject engagement with a capitalist system—and in fact hoped that it might bring them new avenues of prosperity. Their concerns about healing were less a reflection of a desire to step completely outside a capitalist system than an enduring preoccupation with money circulating in socially and morally appropriate ways—as accumulation was often combined with enduring practices of gifting and exchange (Tassi 2017; Yampara et al. 2007). Skepticism of healers who had become overly commodified, I suggest, also highlighted how the body itself could be an especially durable site for preoccupations about ruptured relations. People continued to worry about illnesses that might come with urbanization, as well as the growing inefficacy of healing.

Yet healers themselves often insisted that they had not become completely alienated from the relations that constituted the core of their practice. Anna Tsing points out that while "things as well as people are alienated under capitalism" (2015, 122), this state of being is not stable. Converting a gift into a commodity requires investments and energies—and at various points in the supply chain, people may work to reconvert commodities into gifts with "relation-making powers"

(124). Many healers understood their practice to retain anti-extractive elements that could be invoked in different moments, in different ways. For ritual healers like Patricio, continuing to sustain life meant highlighting how the provision of medicinal remedies remained tied to enduring relations with earth beings. For naturistas, in turn, this often meant emphasizing the connections between the commodity and a more natural, landed past. For both, it often meant emphasizing more long-term, attentive relations of care that they could provide when bio-medical providers could not. Healers positioned the commodities they produced as things that could never be fully alienated—and that might, in fact, heal the ills of labor precarity, exploitation, and alienation in urban contexts.

Emphasizing the enduring centrality of life-making relations for their practice, healers pointed out that a central barrier to healing was not their own commodification, but the lack of support from state, medical, and nonprofit institutions. Patricio, for example, described how he used to prepare herbal poultices to heal broken bones, because children would injure themselves while playing. "Now it must be the same," he speculated, referring to the fact that children were especially subject to these kinds of injuries. "But I don't know. I'm not paid." Patricio quickly moved from his concerns that he was no longer as tuned in to what kinds of ailments were common to his concern about noncompensation; linking the two, he implied that the latter concern was responsible for the former. If patients sometimes worried that healers had become less efficacious because they were not enacting the right relations, many healers worried that state institutions were not enacting the right relations toward them. That is, institutions were not always enacting ethical circulations of money that might both materially and ontologically sustain healing practice.

DOUBLE BINDS OF LABOR

I had known Patricio for several months when he began talking about the impossibility of work in the hospital. One morning in 2015, I joined him as he sat on a ledge just inside the main entrance to the Machacamarca Hospital, underneath a large board that showed the weekly schedule for hospital staff shifts. On the board, the names of traditional medical practitioners and midwives had been inserted into the schedule alongside the names of doctors in primary care, emergency care, and specialties like gynecology and pediatrics.

All that morning, Patricio had been quietly watching patients file past him as they lined up to get appointment slips for the day; occasionally, he talked to patients he knew. Speaking in a mix of Spanish and Aymara, he grumbled to me that patients rarely came to see him in the hospital. Town residents preferred to call him on his cellphone so that he would come see them in their homes. "Here, I almost never treat *sobreparto* or *susto* because I go to people's homes," he sighed, naming two illnesses common in the rural Andes. Sobreparto was an illness resulting from cold temperatures or lack of good relations during childbirth, whereas susto entailed sickness induced by fright. "If they do come to the hospital, I have to tell them I will come to them another day. Here, no, *pues*," Patricio muttered. "Where could I treat these things? Or give massages? The only thing I can give here are teas, these prepared teas, I prescribe them."

Healers I interviewed frequently expressed their desires to work in the hospital, but often found it to be a limited space for enacting their practice. Patricio worried that the only kinds of remedy he could bring into the hospital were portable commodities that he had prepared at home, and that the hospital's lack of support made it difficult for him to practice the full range of healing in his repertoire. His frustration reflected how more commodified forms of healing had been easier to incorporate into institutional settings—but also how state, medical, and nonprofit institutions more broadly had failed to provide material support for his practice. Echoing Reynaldo's earlier words, Patricio directed my attention during our conversation to the wilting greenhouse and to the threadbare consultorio that had been allotted to the hospital's traditional healers, noting that it was not well stocked, and he often had to bring his own supplies.

His frustrations prompted him to wonder whether working in the hospital was worth it. "Here, we have been working so long, but we don't receive a salary," he sighed. "It should be guaranteed, but that's how it is for us. So, I keep working. Sometimes, I think, 'Should I just leave?' But then I think, 'No.'"

Patricio was not the only healer to express frustrations with the lack of pay and yet still decide to continue working in the hospital. Despite their criticisms, healers continued to show up to their regular shifts in part because they saw maintaining a presence in the hospital as important for establishing their legitimacy, particularly given the past criminalization of their practice. Showing up for shifts and adopting other bureaucratic markers (such as submitting patients' records and obtaining official credentials) became a way to shore up their position in a precarious economic context while also generating new possibilities for reinventing themselves as modern practitioners, on a par with biomedical doctors. In other words, these actions were strategic, but also central to how healers sought to reimagine themselves and their practice. In fact, access to credentials and ability to work in public clinics and hospitals had been a key demand of traditional healing activists as they pushed for the passing of the Law of Traditional and Ancestral Medicine. At the same time, adopting these bureaucratic markers became a way to enter into relation with and render themselves visible to state and medical institutions in new ways; they hoped that if they actively participated in these forms, institutional actors might also reciprocate with eventual compensation and other forms of material support.[12]

In the hope that they might be able to leverage redistributive claims on dominant institutions, healers also participated actively in spaces of political representation. As I described in Chapter 1, many healers initially organized to advocate for the legalization of their practice under the auspices of the CSUTCB, an organization that emerged in the 1970s as an alternative to state-sponsored peasant unions (Álvarez Quispe and Loza 2014; Burman 2017). After legalization—and especially after neoliberal multicultural and popular participation reforms were enacted in the 1990s—organizations representing healers proliferated (Babis 2018), echoing other widespread forms of associational life in Bolivia that bridged labor organizing with civil society claims-making

(Albro 2010). Under the new Law of Traditional and Ancestral Medicine enacted in 2013, all healers (regardless of whether they worked in a clinical setting) were required to join a local *consejo* (council) of healers—or form one if it did not already exist. The Machacamarca council of traditional healers had only recently formed at the time of my research in 2015. It had about twenty members from the town and surrounding villages, including but not limited to practitioners who worked in the hospital. The Morales administration promoted such organizations with the stated goal of granting a central role to grassroots organizations in health policy implementation. At the same time, state officials also hoped that such organizations would play a key role in regulating themselves (see Hummel 2021). Healer organizations were charged with ensuring that their members were qualified healers and with submitting paperwork to regional and national health offices so that their members could obtain official credentials.

In Bolivia, larger labor and grassroots organizations often held considerable political power. Yet joining one of the institutionally mandated organizations for healers could be a complicated space for political claims-making. Healer unions did not have the size or political weight that other formal and informal worker unions in Bolivia had to call a strike or mount a road blockade. And while participating in these organizations was required under new legislation, healers' demands could also be received with skepticism by state officials.

One morning in late 2014, I met with Ramón, the sociologist and bureaucrat at the Ministry of Health mentioned in Chapter 1, who worked on implementing the Morales administration's SAFCI policy. He had grown increasingly frustrated with complaints from healing unions about the shortcomings of decolonial health policies. "There is a bit of confusion coming from traditional medicine—that is, from the traditional doctor unions, who think that the SAFCI is the opportunity for them to enter the health care system in a salaried way," he remarked as we sat for an interview in his office. "It's a syndical demand, very union-based, very *salarialista* [salary-oriented]. This is a big problem that we have."

He paused and then backtracked, hedging his prior words. "We believe in articulation and complementarity [between medicines], and we believe that traditional healers should be economically recognized, of course—but not all of them, nor in every place," he continued. "In rural areas, healers are not interested in going to the health center to waste their time. But it does interest healers in peri-urban and urban areas, who have already been making their economic life from traditional healing."

In raising concerns about healers' demands for compensation, Ramón foregrounded divides between different kinds of healers— between rural healers outside the market economy and more urbanized healers, who increasingly made a living by practicing out of private consultorios and selling medicinal plant commodities. In drawing divides between different kinds of healers, Ramón broadly echoed the concerns of some Machacamarqueños, who considered commodification to be antithetical to effective healing. But Ramón also leveraged these concerns in ways that deflected from demands for compensation and suggested that unions were inauthentically representing healer perspectives by being too "salary oriented." In doing so, he also sidestepped how new national laws in fact required all healers (regardless of their preference) to obtain national credentials, join a union, and certify their practice. He also sidestepped how healers demanding compensation were precisely those who were already working within the formal health care system.

While Ramón was more skeptical of healer union demands, most Bolivian health officials I interviewed agreed that, in principle, healers should be paid for their labor. They proposed that municipal governments should cover local healers' salaries, much as they covered some of the salaries of biomedical practitioners working in local health establishments. However, in practice, municipal governments also had limited budgets and rarely provided for healer salaries. In short, while bureaucrats at multiple levels of government broadly agreed on the need for compensation, they gave the issue low priority and never instated a plan to ensure consistent compensation for healers working in public institutions. Over the course of my research, only one highland municipality out of twelve that I visited had allocated funds to pay healers. Amid these shortages, officials suggested that healers who worked in public hospitals should charge patients directly for their services, rather than having patients pay the set consultation fee to the hospital (see also Loza 2008). However, hospital administrators worried about traditional practitioners being able to charge separate, nonstandard fees that could also put an increased financial burden on patients.

The low priority given to the question of healer compensation echoed wider trends in global health policymaking, in which traditional and alternative medical practitioners have been mobilized to perform un- or undercompensated labor in the service of formal health care systems. In the wake of the 1978 Alma Ata Accords, the WHO encouraged the integration of traditional medical practitioners into formal health care services, with the idea that they could help build community trust and also serve as low-cost labor to fill in gaps in underresourced health systems (Langwick 2008)—a dynamic that also intensified in many places after neoliberal structural adjustment made further cuts to state spending on health care (Janes 1999).[13] Bolivian policymakers distanced themselves from other regional and global health policies by emphasizing the need to fully recognize traditional medicine on its own terms, on an equal footing with biomedicine (see Chapter 1). Yet the low priority given to healer compensation also revealed the gaps in the Morales administration's redistributive projects, as it formally rejected neoliberalism but remained haunted by it. In practice, they replicated many of the same patterns that positioned healers as supplementary and devalued labor within health care economies.

I argue that the divides that Ramón put forward, as well as the wider devaluing of healer care, reflected wider ways that healers were put into a liminal position within the formal health care system. Even as they expected healers to comply with bureaucratic regulations (such as obtaining credentials, maintaining patients' records, and working in shifts in hospital settings) policymakers often positioned healers' practices as incompatible with modern regimes of knowledge and labor. Bolivian intercultural health policies echoed other double binds of recognition politics that have pitted Indigenous cultural authenticity against the accumulation of wealth (Cattelino 2010).[14] I suggest that in positioning authentic healing as outside regimes of compensation, policymakers also took up long-standing ontological constructions of what constitutes "real" or "productive" labor under capitalism. Scholars have noted that framings of what counts as productive or rational labor have been steeped in racialized hierarchies between humans, as well as between humans and other-than-human entities. The presumed ability to undertake transformative labor—including productive use of land—was central to Enlightenment constructions of the human as white European man, to the exclusion of Indigenous, Black, and subaltern populations (Wynter 2003). Simultaneously, dominant colonial constructions positioned productive labor over the land—and abandonment of Indigenous relations with land—as ostensible pathways for entry into the category of the human (Jackson 2012). These historically rooted regimes continued to haunt not only the devaluation of Indigenous labor itself, but also assumptions that healing, based in ostensibly nonproductive relations with land, did not count as labor at all. Institutional actors associated authentic forms of healing primarily with spiritual relations with land—glossing these as fixed Indigenous "cultural beliefs"—and in doing so, positioned it as outside the realm of compensation.

These double binds—in which healers were expected to comply with dominant regimes of labor and yet were also deemed incompatible with them—trickled their way into daily forms of bureaucratic regulation and assessment of healing practice. On the one hand, the Law of Traditional and Ancestral Medicine instated measures for regulating, professionalizing, and credentialing healers—a demand that had come from healer activist movements hoping to gain increasing legitimacy for their practice. Healers were required to submit extensive paperwork to the ministry to obtain their official credentials from the government—including records of having attended training courses, community testimonials that they were a real healer, and lists of specific patients and medications they had prescribed. Healers, like those in the Machacamarca Hospital, who worked for the formal health care system were also required to show up for regular shifts and submit their patient records to the Ministry of Health (including for patients they saw on their own outside the hospital).

On the other hand, state officials, NGO workers, and hospital administrators often assumed that healers (at least in their more authentic iterations) practiced forms of knowledge that were fundamentally separate from biomedicine—and from modern rationality more broadly. While policy documents often accounted for a range of healing specialties (one I saw listed thirty different specialties with which healers could identify), they often worked from the presupposition that healers treated problems distinct from biomedicine. With the goal of promoting interculturality in health care, a system of "referral and counter-referral" required that traditional healers refer patients to a biomedical practitioner when a patient had a biomedical problem, while biomedical practitioners would refer patients with culture-bound ailments to traditional healers. Yet when I helped Mariela, a GHA staffer, collect the hospital healers' patient records to send to the Ministry of Health, she expressed surprise that most of the problems listed were metabolic ailments like kidney disease and diabetes, rather than kharikhari, sobreparto, and susto. Binary framings between traditional and modern, nonbiomedical and biomedical knowledge sidestepped how healers—particularly as they moved through a capitalist, urbanized economy—were increasingly treating a range of illnesses, including those that overlapped with biomedical categories (Ramírez Hita 2008). Instead, like many other policies to incorporate traditional healers into health care systems, they often worked from fixed presuppositions of what constituted the "traditional" (Pigg 1996; 1997).

These double binds, in turn, had contradictory effects for how traditional healing was incorporated into hospital settings. Overall, it was easier for healers like naturistas, who already had undergone training and certification programs and who had commodified much of their practice, to demonstrate their compatibility with dominant regulatory systems. As Patricio noted, it was easier to bring prepared, commodified remedies into the hospital setting. At the same time, being perceived as too close to biomedicine or too "salary-oriented" could make one subject to accusations of inauthenticity. Healers were expected to simultaneously comply with modern regimes of knowledge and labor, even as institutional actors often assumed healers' cultural practices to exist outside of these regimes.

In contrast to parteras, who were expected to offer racialized and feminized psychological support during hospital births (see Chapter 3), healers had a less defined role within the hospital. Healers were expected to keep to regular shifts, and they were given an empty exam room where they could see patients. But they also did not work alongside biomedical doctors. Within the formal system of referral and counter-referral, healers expressed some willingness to coordinate with biomedical providers. At the same time, biomedical providers tended to assume that all ailments were biomedical ailments, and so would not refer patients to traditional healers at all. As Patricio reflected, in practice most patients preferred to seek out healers outside the hospital, in their homes or in the healers' private offices. He attributed this to the lack of material sustenance and support healers were provided in the hospital. But Segundo pointed out that many patients also avoided the hospital because they associated the space with a lack of care. He explained, "Some patients I know here go over to my [private] consultorio because in the hospital, you have to wait all morning to see a doctor and the care is not good. They tell me, 'The doctor gave me these medications, and it did not help me.'" If some residents of Machacamarca treated commodified forms of healing with skepticism, many others still saw it as retaining personalized relations of care that were often foreclosed in the hospital setting.

Intercultural health policies were designed to culturally include traditional healers in health care settings. Policymakers positioned healers as recipients of the state's warm care, even as they hoped that healers might extend warm care to patients by helping them feel like their own understandings of health were represented in institutional settings. Yet the same relational care practices that made healers the subjects of cultural inclusion were deemed incompatible with dominant regimes of labor and capitalism. As I have shown, for patients, healers, and other residents of Machacamarca, entry into a capitalist market economy could also provoke anxiety, ambivalence, and debate given its potential rupture of relations considered essential for healing. Yet healers (as well as their patients) also creatively engaged in multiple practices, shifting between market and nonmarket forms as they navigated enduring conditions of precarity and sought to affirm the role of relationality in their healing. In contrast, when they emphasized healers' incompatibility with dominant regimes of knowledge and labor, policymakers solidified racialized constructions of the human that precluded healers from the realm of compensation. Healers sometimes sought to participate in these dominant regimes by keeping to shifts, obtaining credentials, participating in unions, and other forms of legitimating their practice and making themselves visible to the state. However, as I show in the following pages, they also articulated claims that exceeded these forms, precisely by turning back to the kinds of human and more-than-human relations that formed the core of their practice.

RESIGNIFYING REDISTRIBUTION

I want to return, here at the end, to the story that opened this chapter: that of Reynaldo walking through the wilted greenhouse, worried that biomedical providers had been ripping the leaves off plants for their own use. Built by GHA in the early 2000s, the greenhouse had been designed to incorporate traditional medical practice into the hospital space. The warm room, filled with plants and heated by a glass roof, disrupted the clinical, laboratory-like architecture of the hospital that had historically been built to hold up scientific modernity and exclude local cultural specificities and practices.

It was also designed with the idea of bringing relations with land and plants into the hospital, echoing other nonprofit initiatives to revive gardening practices among rural-to-urban migrants. Greenhouses were a newer technology on the Bolivian Altiplano. Several Bolivian NGOs and foundations had invested in greenhouses and gardens in urban areas to help rural-to-urban migrants grow vegetables on small plots in their yards (Farthing and Romer 2019). Several families I knew in Machacamarca had also built greenhouses on their own as a method of growing crops that did not typically grow in the dry, cold climate of the Altiplano. They consumed the crops themselves or sold them on the market.

Historically, healers had not grown their own plants in gardens, as they usually harvested them in the wild or bought dried plants at the market. But many healers expressed their enthusiasm for the greenhouse as a way to assert their presence and belonging in a space where they had often been excluded. The garden also created a space for experimenting with new kinds of relations with plants—one that also further established healing as a non-alienated, life-sustaining practice. Yet if healers expressed some optimism about possibilities of the greenhouse, they also expressed frustration about its deterioration—which they saw as connected to wider conditions of extraction and lack of material support for healers in the hospital.

Gardens could be complex spaces that shifted between sustaining and denying conditions of flourishing. For many anthropologists writing about small-scale gardens and greenhouses, such spaces have important potential for cultivating relations otherwise and challenging conditions of dispossession, scarcity, and exploitation (Garcia 2010; Langwick 2018; Reese 2019). As Stacey Langwick argues, alternative medicine projects like medicinal plant gardens are not pristine spaces; they do not exist in a pure state outside of dominant systems. Nonetheless, through collaborative and patchy processes of decomposition and growth, they "intervene into relationships between plants and people— re-making them in ways that unsettle assemblages built through colonial plantations, national development, and extractive capital" (2018, 417). Others, however, have demonstrated how gardens, greenery, and similar projects designed around progressive goals of ecological flourishing can also operate as central sites of racial inequality and exploitation of a largely volunteer labor force in which conditions of noncompensation are often justified in the name of working toward a moral, ecological good (Maurer 2020; Randle 2022).

What began as a hopeful project of reestablishing relations quickly folded back into the dynamics of conscripting free labor that already unfolded in the hospital space. As GHA staffers were frequently on the road during the day—visiting projects and health centers throughout the region—they could not always maintain the greenhouse space themselves and had difficulty finding someone who could do it. Plants were unruly, and they required daily attention. And they ultimately required the conscription of voluntary labor in this work of care. Staffers asked the hospital groundskeeper to water and weed the plants regularly, but he was also consumed with other tasks required to maintain the rest of the hospital space. They then asked the healers to do it, but the healers were already unwaged and likewise consumed with other work, in and out of the hospital. Noting that I was at the hospital nearly every day, the staffers asked me to do it for a while, and so I did.

Amid shifting conditions of labor and maintenance, the greenhouse cycled through various phases of repair and disrepair, of growth and of deterioration. Shortly before an event on intercultural health, in which Ministry of Health officials and representatives from other major NGOs were set to visit the Machacamarca hospital, GHA staffers made sure to trim the plants and put in freshly painted signs (Figure 4.1). They also asked the healers to help prepare a display of dried medicinal plants with labels to mount on a table in the greenhouse (Figure 4.2). Staffers wanted to demonstrate to the ministry and other NGOs that intercultural health projects were working.

But such moments also highlighted for healers what possibilities institutional investments might enable, were they to be more consistent. Institutional sustenance might include money and compensation—and it might also include investments in material infrastructures and plants that healers used to cultivate ties essential to healing and care. Healers hoped to reconnect people to land-based relations, but argued that state, medical, and nonprofit institutions also needed to participate in these relations to cultivate the conditions of flourishing.

One morning in the hospital, I attended a meeting of the municipal healers' union in which GHA staffers had invited an agronomy student from a university in La Paz to consult with healers about new plants to put in the greenhouse. Noting the same state of disrepair that Rey-

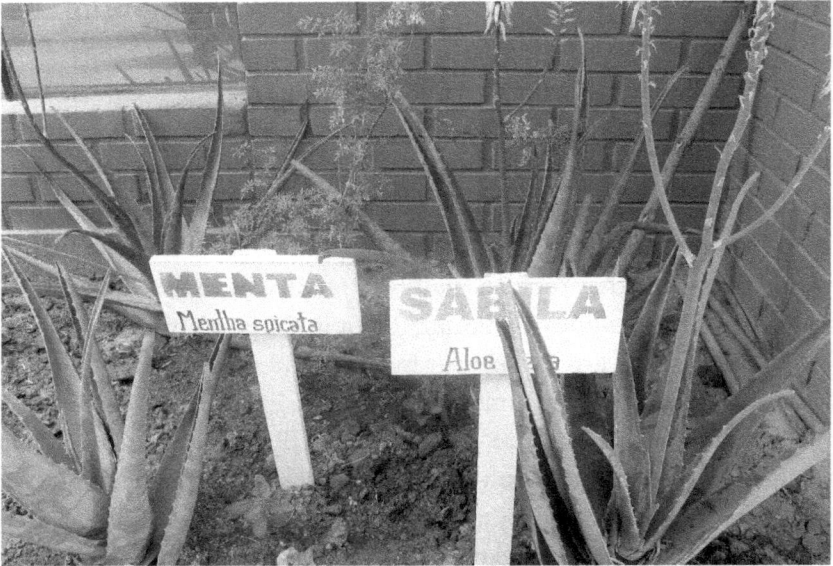

FIGURE 4.1. The greenhouse in the Machacamarca Hospital, in advance of a visit from state and NGO officials. GHA installed freshly painted signs and trimmed and replaced several of the plants. Source: Photograph by the author.

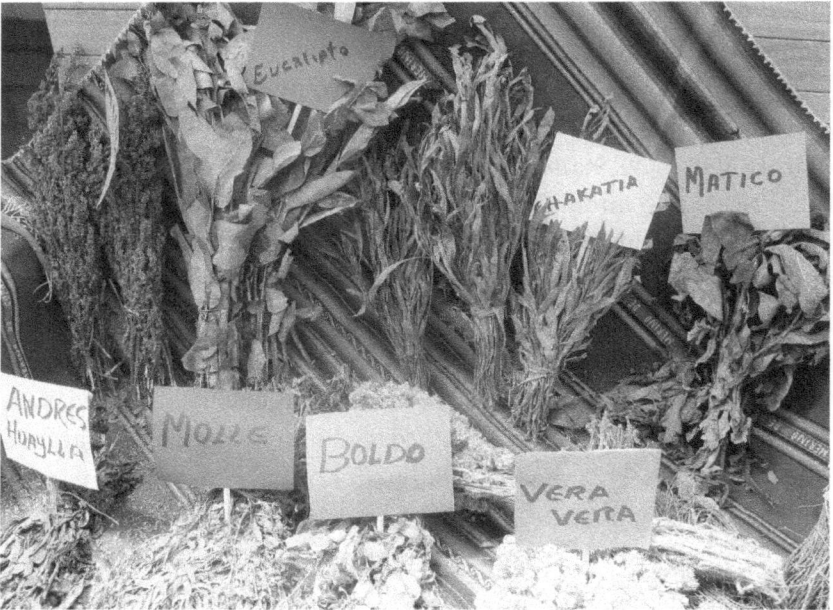

FIGURE 4.2. A display of medicinal plants, prepared by the hospital healers. Source: Photograph by the author.

naldo had described as we walked through the greenhouse together, the NGO staffers had recruited students to remove dead medicinal plants and put in new ones. Healers jumped on the opportunity to ask for investments in the space that might facilitate their practice.

When the agronomy student asked the healers what medicinal plants they wanted in the greenhouse, healers immediately suggested coca. The coca plant had long been central to ritual, medicinal, and communal practices in the Andes. It did not typically grow in the climate of the Altiplano but had historically been brought to the region through circuits of exchange with communities living on the Andean semitropical slopes where it did grow.

For healers and many other people living in Machacamarca, the coca plant facilitated social relationships (Allen 2002; Spedding 1997). It was common during gatherings (ranging from political events to family gatherings) for someone to bring a bag of coca to pass around and share. Coca was also brewed in teas and chewed during the workday to facilitate labor—the grassy leaves turning one's spit green and helping stave off effects of hunger and altitude. Patricio and other ritual healers had long used coca leaves to divine the future. They also made offerings of coca (for example, by blowing leaves or burning *k'oas*) to cultivate relations of care with earth beings and ensure their guardianship (Allen 2002; de la Cadena 2015). As urbanization appeared to threaten relations with earth beings, Patricio sought nonetheless to sustain these relations; he continued to regularly visit the hilltops and make offerings using coca leaves.

For naturistas, coca again took a different relational form. Evangelical churches condemned the preparation of coca leaf offerings to earth beings and sometimes even condemned the regular chewing of the coca leaf (Salas Carreño 2019). But naturistas did not entirely reject coca, nor its facilitation of social relationships in a community. They did not make offerings with coca, but often continued to chew it. They used it as the basis for numerous teas, tonics, pomades, and other remedies. Within the past few decades, coca had also increasingly become commercialized throughout Bolivia, the driver of numerous pharmaceutical cottage industries (Sikkink 2010). But for naturistas in

Machacamarca, coca, much like other plants, continued to be effective precisely because of its ties with the imaginary of an ancestral landed past. Coca remedies became a way to reestablish relations that had been ruptured and consume them in a new form.

Significantly, coca had also become a central symbol of the Morales administration's decolonial project. The MAS—a political party that had emerged out of coca-growing unions—had decriminalized the production of the leaf. Rhetorically, it emphasized the importance of coca to Indigenous practice and identity and rejected international drug enforcement narratives that primarily associated the leaf with the production of cocaine. The Morales administration expelled the U.S. Drug Enforcement Agency that had brought violence on coca producers in the Yungas and Chaparre regions. It created a Ministry of Coca as it was also increasingly investing in domestic coca products, such as coca flour, liquor, candy, and pharmaceuticals (Grisaffi 2019). The coca leaf, then, brought together multiple threads: it was both a central entity in their healing practice and a central symbol of the state's own promises of decolonization.

And yet, when the healers made the suggestion to replant the greenhouse with coca, the agronomy student countered that it was a bad idea. She explained that coca leached too many nutrients from the soil, and it would affect the other plants in the greenhouse. In doing so, she echoed environmentalist discourses that had positioned the rapid growth of coca as environmentally destructive and as taking over other, more sustainable crops. In the student's narrative of extraction, coca could leach other plants; it could contribute to challenges of maintaining the liveliness of the greenhouse. The student's framing—ultimately supported by the NGO—was ontologically distinct from what healers experienced to be the source of leaching: the lack of pay and material investment. Healers disagreed that the coca was a harmful or leaching plant. For them, extraction stemmed not from the plant itself but from institutions that had not followed through on obligations.

In asking for the greenhouse to be replanted with coca, they were in part asking institutions to invest in plants as they did before official events, when the greenhouse became vibrant and lush once again. But they also hoped that institutions might participate in and facilitate the relations central to their healing practice, particularly in a context of enduring precarity for both them and their patients. Calling on institutions to plant coca was more than symbolic; it pulled the state into different kinds of life-making relations, particularly in a context where many felt those ties had been ruptured by urbanization. Flows of institutional funds could repair relations and sustain healing both through material effects (purchasing more alive plants, paying for the maintenance of the greenhouse) and their relational, ontological effects (reflecting the kinds of moral practice essential to corporeal well-being). Even as these demands were limited and not always heard, they reflected how healers attempted to rework institutional projects to craft different configurations of redistribution.

For James Ferguson (2015), state redistributive policies (such as universal basic income or cash transfer programs) offer possibilities for moving beyond the idea that salaried labor—or what he and Tania Li (2018) call "the proper job"—will inherently bring economic development. In a late capitalist era when jobs are increasingly precarious, contingent, or simply nonexistent, state redistribution might offer an alternative route to ensuring that people across the board are able to live dignified lives (Ferguson 2015). In asking institutions to engage in gifting and redistributive relations, healers challenged racialized regimes of labor and compensation that had largely precluded them from the category of productive work; instead, they positioned institutions as having a wider moral obligation to care for bodies and lands in a precarious world.

But in doing so, healers also problematized universalizing models of redistribution: those, like the revolutionary government after 1952, that largely ignored questions of Indigeneity or racial inequality—or those, like the Morales administration, that continued to pit cultural recognition against redistribution, despite promises to bring these two approaches together. Instead, ontologies of healing and the body as constituted through relations became a central ground for articulating claims and setting the terms of material redistribution. In making claims situated in corporeal and land-based relations, healers echoed what influential Aymara political theorist Fausto Reinaga argued in his work: that rather than look to Eurocentric models of socialism, Indigenous people might theorize their own alternatives to colonialism and capitalism, based in their own practices of reciprocity and redistribution (1969). Yet where Reinaga primarily looked to a more pristine rural past outside the context of urbanization, healers engaged in heterogeneous practices that reasserted forms of life-making as they moved in and out of capitalist forms. The coca plant took on multiple meanings: a commodity that might be bought and sold on the market, a central actor in the cultivation of healing relations, and a site where institutions might also potentially nurture these relations. In a context in which alienation (resulting from urbanization and the state's exploitation of healer labor) was a growing concern, healers hoped that institutional investments might facilitate new forms of care.

In 2013, at a health fair in the capital city of La Paz, I met Teodora and Ismael, two healers from a village a couple of hours' drive from Machacamarca but located in a different municipality and health district. The fair, sponsored by the La Paz Departmental Health Service, had numerous stands ranging from vaccination booths to educational information on health prevention. With some support from GHA staffers, who provided funding for the tent and for a spot in the fair, the two healers set up a stand where they sold pomades in small white plastic jars and tins, prepared in a laboratory that had been attached to their local health center. I asked Teodora and Ismael if I could interview them, and we sat there and chatted, occasionally pausing the interview when a customer showed up to buy pomades. During our conversation, Teodora and Ismael described feeling supported: unlike healers in many other districts, they were paid a salary by their local government.

Some weeks later, I accompanied GHA to a site visit in Teodora and Ismael's village. I met the healers again as they showed us around their traditional medicine laboratory. The laboratory had been built with funds from GHA and was one of three in the La Paz Department that was in the process of being formally accredited. The small room was lined with shelves full of dried plants, bottles, and processed pomades. In the corner sat a cooktop for preparing the remedies.

Creating an apparatus for healers to produce commodities for sale did not resolve all the tensions involved with incorporating healing into the hospital; healers continued to face an uphill battle for recognition and worried that commodification could still impede effective healing. Yet institutional investment and material support also enabled new possibilities of care that were not available to healers in Machacamarca and, indeed, in many parts of Bolivia.

In ending with this encounter with Teodora and Ismael, I highlight possibilities of redistribution—however imperfect—through which healers might feel sustained. Despite the adoption of activist frameworks of relational health and radical pluralism, policies remained constrained both by ongoing resource shortages and by enduring ontological hierarchies, ultimately deprioritizing pay and material support for healers. As a result, Bolivian state policies put healers in a liminal position when bringing them in to work for the formal health care system.

Yet healers themselves framed redistribution from the state as facilitating their ability to nourish patients' well-being. As healers grappled with conditions of exploitation, they redefined state material distribution as a question of caring for relations. By situating noncompensation as part of a broader pattern of alienation, healers situated a lack of material sustenance within wider concerns about urbanization in the wake of structural adjustment. If Teodora and Ismael had been able to obtain material support that they found helpful, healers in Machacamarca often had more difficulty getting their demands heard. And yet, their ongoing participation in the hospital space and bureaucratic credentialing highlighted how they continually sought to hold institutions accountable to their obligations, in the hopes of creating more habitable worlds.

5 DOCTOR, PATIENT, KIN

Remaking Hospital Relations

EARLY ONE MORNING, I JOINED a small group of GHA staffers and hospital biomedical practitioners as they gathered at a small health post in a village a short drive from the town of Machacamarca and still located within the same municipality. The small, two-room post was staffed by a single auxiliary nurse, Rubén, who greeted the group as they filed into his office. The goal for the day was to complete household surveys known as *carpetas familiares* (family files) for the households in the district served by the health post.

The carpetas were a central component of health policy efforts under Evo Morales to systematically facilitate biomedical practitioners' knowledge of social determinants of health in the wider community they were serving. For practitioners working in health posts in more remote rural areas, their work had already for decades depended on household visits—for example, as they administered vaccinations or assisted in complicated home births. The carpetas, however, were designed to make household visits more systematic and oriented around the collection of data on social determinants in the community. In turn, for practitioners based in larger clinics and hospitals, who usually treated patients when they came into the hospital rather than in their homes, the carpetas were also designed to help them meet community members and understand health problems in the district.

Because the Machacamarca Hospital served the entire municipality, a handful of interns from the hospital had come to help Rubén complete the surveys for the villages in his district, as one person could not complete the job alone. Yet, with a deadline to submit the household data to the Ministry of Health looming, it was unclear that even the mobilization of the hospital labor force would be sufficient. Going from door to door and filling out the carpetas, as I came to learn, was time-consuming work. In more isolated rural areas, especially, completing surveys often involved traveling long distances between houses and crossing large expanses of farm fields. With the goal of helping to implement national policies, GHA staffers volunteered to help complete the surveys, joining forces with Rubén and the hospital interns to cover more ground. They divvied up the labor, so that each group of surveyors would cover a different village served by the health post.

Two GHA staffers, Elena and Mariela, invited me to join their group, so I tagged along as we walked back to the white NGO truck parked outside the health post. They had been assigned to a village that was furthest from the health post, as they were the only group with a vehicle for transport. Samuel, the NGO's staff driver, took us down a dirt road that cut a straight, narrow line through fields of quinoa and alfalfa on the Bolivian Altiplano. Despite the early hour, the sun was already beating down, creating a contrast between yellow fields and bright blue sky. Finally, the white GHA truck stopped in front of a mud-brick house at the edge of a village. An older man—his face weathered from the sun, his sweater and pants flecked with dust—was raking up hay for the large black cows standing at a distance. He set down his rake and looked at us curiously as the truck pulled up in front of him.

Mariela, one of the GHA staffers, got out of the truck and greeted him. Shaking the man's hand, she told him she and her colleagues were helping providers from the nearby hospital fill out household surveys for each of the households in his village. She asked if he would be willing to answer some questions.

The man, named Paulino, sat down on a bushel of hay and nodded in agreement. I was holding the stack of blank Ministry of Health survey forms, and Mariela took one from me. Penciling in answers with some difficulty—as she had no hard surface on which to write—she asked Paulino about who else lived in his household. Then, she went through a lengthy list of questions: How many people sleep in each room of your house? How do you dispose of waste? How much grain, meat, fruits and vegetables, oil, and iodized salt do you consume every day? Does anyone in your family have an illness? Do you ever visit traditional healers?

Like many village residents we would meet that day, Paulino responded to each question in a way that emphasized his use of biomedicine and his preoccupation with health and hygiene. His family ate a varied and healthy diet, he insisted. He never went to see a traditional healer.

———

Carpetas familiares were a central component of Bolivian Ministry of Health projects to factor social determinants of health into the provision of care. As I described in Chapter 1, ministry officials I interviewed emphasized the importance of shedding asistencialismo, or strictly treatment-based care, in favor of more expansive, family- and community-based methods of illness prevention and health promotion. Bolivian policymakers drew from wider regional and global health frameworks that positioned attention to social determinants as a way to move beyond a focus on the individual and attend to structural and socioeconomic factors that underpinned health (Yates-Doerr 2020). At the same time, Bolivian policymakers explicitly couched community-based approaches to health as stemming from Indigenous cosmologies of well-being, situated in relations with "family, community, and nature" (Ministerio de Salud y Deportes 2008, 20, my translation). Policy texts treated social determinants frameworks and Indigenous ontologies of health as fundamentally compatible, even interchangeable, given that both approaches centered social relations beyond the individual body as the basis for health.

In this chapter, I trace how surveys of local households both facilitated and foreclosed the provision of care. The carpetas bureaucratized and systematized the more informal household visits that had once been central to rural health work. Providers conducted surveys and then drew community risk maps based on the data they collected, coming to visualize and care for the community as a whole in terms of broader risk patterns. While scholars have often focused on bureaucracy's production of indifference and anonymity (Herzfeld 1993; Stevenson 2014), I show how both state officials and biomedical providers saw the surveys as another modality of warm care—one that enabled renewed attention to patient conditions and needs.

At the same time, the carpetas as a mechanism of care through data collection ultimately reentrenched colonial biopolitical paradigms that located risk within Indigenous household and kinship relations. Paulino, for instance, was asked how much iodized salt he consumed, or how many people slept in a room in his household. And he responded in ways that lined up with dominant biomedical models of health—by insisting, for example, that he always ate a healthy diet. As the survey racialized medical risk by associating it primarily with rural Indigenous practices, many respondents like Paulino answered in ways that aligned with dominant biomedical framings and expectations. I suggest that the surveys' approach to documenting health risk reflected the stickiness of colonial categories through projects of transformation, as well as how bureaucratic data collection practices themselves fix bodies and relations in place.

The surveys' location of risk ultimately ignored—and sometimes hindered—long-standing moral norms of rural health care, in which Indigenous Aymara patients sought to bring providers into relations of patronage and godparenting to facilitate healing. For many patients, kinship extended beyond biological ties and brought medical providers into the very relations that sustained well-being. In Machacamarca and surrounding villages, people often sought to bring providers into relations of material exchange and *compadrazgo* (ritual co-parenting) to facilitate healing. Echoing forms of patronage and clientelism elsewhere in Latin America, compadrazgo often involved asking someone with relatively greater resources or a relatively greater position of power to become kin (sometimes called "vertical compadrazgo") (Mintz and Wolf 1950). In the Andes, specifically, compadrazgo involved building long-term kin relations, not only between godparents and godchildren but also parents and godparents, who referred to each other as *comadre* (co-mother) and *compadre* (co-father) (Leinaweaver 2008; Van Vleet 2008). In the context of medical care-seeking in Machacamarca, compadrazgo facilitated new forms of ethical accountability from providers and transformed conditions of care. Bound by ties of compadrazgo, patients might call upon providers to fulfill their obligations at various, as-yet undefined points in the future, not just at a singular point of illness.

Carpetas, designed to cultivate new forms of attention and relation with families and communities, largely positioned providers as operating outside the relations that constituted health and well-being. Instead, kinship was rendered legible primarily as a site of risk and intervention. In tracing survey practices, I continue to examine how Bolivian policy engagements with Indigenous knowledges and modes of relation reentrenched a colonial biopolitics. At the same time, attention to localized practices of kinship and relationality points to how patients continually reworked dominant medical systems toward different ends of care. Kin-making, as Kim TallBear suggests, might also offer a basis for different modes of recognition (beyond those posed by the liberal settler state) and become a key site for Indigenous agency to decide who might become part of a community (cited in Tuck 2016; see also Winchell 2022, 13). As Mareike Winchell (2022) argues, such non-normative modes of kinship in Bolivia enable forms of ethical intimacy and accountability beyond dominant framings of the nuclear family. Choosing kin, in this instance, became a means to tackle the indifference and uncertainty of state care and hold individual practitioners accountable to their patients. As patients drew practitioners into relations of ethical obligation, moreover, they destabilized and reshaped the terms of state care and biopolitical intervention. I end by asking how patients' moves to bring providers into kin networks shifted relations away from being construed as a site of risk and toward positioning them as a dynamic in which providers were also imbricated.

MAKING KIN IN RURAL HEALTH CARE

For many of my interlocutors who were residents of Machacamarca, kinship ties with providers had long shaped the trajectories of medical care. Before the construction of larger institutions like the Machacamarca municipal hospital, rural health care provision historically relied on practitioners providing care to patients in their homes. Nurses would often work out of one-room health posts. They would travel to households in the community when undertaking health education and vaccination campaigns, as well as when patients called them to treat a specific health problem. In conversations, Machacamarqueños recalled when the first health post had been constructed in the area in the 1960s. Attached to the railway station that at the time provided the main source of traffic through the rural town, the health post was staffed by a single nurse. Years later, people still recalled the nurse with fondness. As one of my elderly neighbors, Timoteo, reminisced, "In the town, the nurse had many compadres. Godchildren as well. He had already won over the town and the communities. [People] went, 'Please, Doctor, cure me, I am sick.'"

Another elderly neighbor, Luciano, similarly brought up the nurse in Machacamarca's first health establishment when I asked him what he remembered about health care services in the past. As we stood in the bright sun in front of his house, he suggested it was people's efforts to bring the nurse into reciprocal relations that had prompted him to attend to them. According to him, "They brought the nurse, and he started. He knew how to inject people. At that time, the rail company had brought him in to treat only the workers. For the people from here, there was nothing. But some of them brought him sugar and milk. He liked that. And so, the medical services expanded. Now, we have *profesionales* working here."

For Luciano, the fact that town residents had brought the nurse sugar and milk—thereby bringing him into a circle of gifting and exchange—directly facilitated healing and even led to the expansion of medical services in town. Both men's recollections pointed to how dynamics of kinship and exchange were built into rural biomedicine from the start, thereby refracting state projects, categories, and modes of authority into existing forms of relation (Han 2012).

Although kinship practices could take many forms, vertical compadrazgo had long been a central means to facilitate relationships across economic and racial hierarchies in Andean regions (Leinaweaver 2008). In Machacamarca, residents asked medical practitioners, anthropologists, schoolteachers, politicians, and even slightly wealthier neighbors to become kin. One might ask others to become godparents for the baptism of a child, but also for significant life events like graduations and weddings. One might even become godparent of an entire graduating class. This meant that both a child and their parents could have multiple kin relations forged through compadrazgo. Like the forms of relationality and moral practice I described in Chapter 4, kin ties were enacted through ritual and material exchange, as families provided godparents with food and drink, and godparents provided gifts and sometimes money. Such practices also sometimes exceeded strict religious affiliations. While Evangelical Protestant converts also developed kin networks through their tight-knit church communities (Lazar 2008, 158), many Evangelicals I met in Machacamarca simultaneously continued to participate in baptisms and engage in forms of compadrazgo.

For scholars working in Bolivia, one central point of concern has been how kin-based modes of social life have been the subject of state and NGO scrutiny and intervention, particularly under projects to sustain liberal models of individual autonomy and freedom. Silvia Rivera Cusicanqui's foundational study of the ayllu in northern Potosí highlights how multiple generations of state and nonprofit reformers have misinterpreted ayllu systems (kin-based systems of communal governance) as threats to liberal democracy; yet, as she emphasizes, "Attempts by liberals, populists, and leftists to impose liberal democratic models on the ayllus have actually hindered the emergence and consolidation of democratic practices and institutions in Bolivian society, reproducing authoritarian and/or paternalistic relations rooted in the colonial and oligarchic past" (1990, 102). Rivera Cusicanqui's work not only highlights the contradictions of liberalism—in which projects undertaken in the name of individual progress and freedom end up reinscribing inequalities—but also reclaims kinship as a key site of Indigenous political practice.[1]

Building from these foundational discussions, two recent anthropological works have revisited the ethical and relational complexities of kinship practices, as well as how these continue to encounter institutional projects of reform. Susan Ellison (2018) examines how compadrazgo and other forms of obligational exchange shape local networks of moneylending among Aymara residents in the city of El Alto. Foregrounding the centrality of relations of reciprocity and exchange to constituting personhood, she highlights how these relations require "material expression and work" (141) that can also be fraught and can move between care and coercion. In this context, "social relations are also taxed by the very practices that constitute them, including widespread informal lending between kin and other social relations" (138). These messy and vital social entanglements come into tension, however, with projects put forward by alternate dispute resolution centers in the city of El Alto. Drawing from a liberal understanding of personhood, center staff members look to frame dispute resolution as a conflict between two autonomous parties, setting aside the complex role of kin and other third parties in debt networks. In doing so, staff members also seek to make what they think of as unwieldy conflicts more manageable.

Mareike Winchell (2022), working with Quechua and mestizo communities in the valleys of Cochabamba, turns to the historical centrality of kin relations between hacienda masters and servants, tracing how these kin relations continue to be enacted among their descendants in the present. In a post-hacienda present, enduring kin attachments are an ethical ground for holding the descendants of hacienda masters accountable to a violent past—thus "reconfiguring oppressive kinds of intimacy as ethical grounds for Indigenous demands for accountability in the present" (37). These modes of relationality, she points out, became problematic for the Morales administration's land reform projects, which framed liberation primarily in terms of individual free labor and property rights.

Drawing from these works, I point to how kinship became a central point of friction in the context of Bolivian health care reforms. Kin arrangements, I suggest, were at the center of competing understandings of health and the body itself. While state officials claimed inspiration from Indigenous relational constructions of well-being, the surveys largely positioned kinship as a site of risk to health. In turn, for many of my interlocutors who were residents of Machacamarca and surrounding villages, kinship ties differently shaped bodily states. I highlight in this chapter how practices of kinship and exchange flowed into the body and facilitated healing; gifts like milk and sugar—and also the obligations that went into them—might build up a well body. These material arrangements sustained the working of biomedicine but also exceeded it. Timoteo described townsfolk actively seeking out the nurse for cures, while Luciano understood exchanges to have contributed to the expansion of biomedical services in town. Yet as my conversations with the two men and with other town residents suggested, people did not fully internalize biomedical models of the body and healing as a result; instead, they reworked biomedical care in ways that aligned with their own approaches to sustaining well-being.

DOCUMENTING KINSHIP

In 2015, I interviewed Delina, a middle-aged mestiza nurse who had been working in the municipal hospital in Machacamarca for three years. Before coming to the hospital, she worked for ten years at a health post in a remote village in the Andes. During our conversation, she described shifts in her practice that occurred with the implementation of the family file system.

> *Delina*: When I started [working at the rural health post], the SAFCI policy did not yet exist. But all the same, we went from house to house, we did health prevention and promotion. Around 2008, I think, when they implemented the SAFCI, they gave us the work of filling out family files. But community-based work always has involved going to people's homes. People really distrust Western

medicine—what we call scientific medicine—so they prefer not to come to the health center and instead cure themselves [at home]. So, one has to try to change this and teach them what is health, also.

Gabriela: What did you do to try to gain their trust?

Delina: People are wary, and it's hard to win them over. One has to treat them with *cariño* [care, affection]. I, for example, tried to be *cariñosa* [caring, affectionate]. I always spoke well to them. They always received me with open doors. But people are wary. When other, new doctors came, people did not want the doctors to treat them. Instead, they sought me out for treatment. So, I talked to them, I showed them, I taught them. So, in that respect, I think I gained their trust.

Gabriela: And when you all started to implement the family files, from the SAFCI policy, did you feel like it was different or similar to what you were already doing?

Delina: We faced similar challenges with the family files. Because in filling out the surveys, [the surveys] ask about the number of people in each family, they ask for various kinds of data. And people are very distrustful of giving out this data. They think that if the data is collected, they might have to pay more taxes, or their lands will be taken. So, for that reason, it was also difficult to convince them.

Delina's words highlighted how rural health work (especially in areas served by smaller health posts and centers) had long involved going from door to door and getting to know members of a community. Like many providers I interviewed, Delina echoed tropes that rural, Indigenous, and campesino patients were inherently suspicious of biomedicine and needed to be taught what constituted "health." At the same time, she foregrounded the time and labor involved in establishing good relations. She suggested that because she had worked in the same community for a long time and had established relations, patients sought her out more frequently than they did newly arrived doctors. From Delina's perspective, the formulation of the SAFCI policy ignored how rural health providers had already been undertaking "health prevention and promotion" and "going to people's homes." Instead, the SAFCI introduced a new technology—the carpetas—that made building good relations more difficult because of surveys' potential associations with state taxation and land dispossession.

Delina's criticisms stuck with me because I knew the carpetas had been designed, in part, with the goal of ensuring that providers were regularly visiting households. In keeping with a social medicine focus, policymakers hoped to move providers outside of the confines of treating patients solely in the clinic—so that they could better engage in preventative care but also so that they could build trust with patients. Health policy texts directly emphasized the importance of strengthening the "interrelation between the personnel providing health services and the people, families, and communities [they served]" (Ministerio de Salud y Deportes 2008, 9, my translation). Household surveys, seemingly, offered a mechanism for making household visits more systematic.

The carpetas were designed to extend state care by making regular visits and data collection the very basis of provider accountability and attention to patient concerns. In Bolivia, as elsewhere, institutions have turned to documentation and quantitative data collection as mechanisms to ensure accountability, transparency, and accuracy.[2] The kinds of personalized care Delina provided—or that Luciano and Timoteo recounted in their reminiscences—were for some bureaucrats and administrators I interviewed too heterogeneous, too subject to a system of personal favors that did not expand care for everyone. Instead, survey data collection would provide a basis for more equitable care across the board. Katherine Mason points to how surveys can also become an important site of what she calls "quantitative care," as population researchers come to care "for, and with, numbers" (2018, 202). For the U.S.-based population researchers she interviewed, the very objectivity of quantitative studies offered a path of moral action; in their view, quantitative studies were a moral means to care at a distance for vulnerable populations that had been treated unjustly. Mason's work helps to illuminate how Bolivian state officials—as well as some of the providers who administered the surveys—understood carpetas to be a mode of extending warm care to patients. If some state reforms were geared toward encouraging providers to adopt warmer, more culturally sensitive approaches inside the clinic (see Chapters 2 and 3), the carpetas were specifically geared to encouraging systematic forms of attention outside the clinic—to ensuring that providers were tuned in to the health concerns of all patients in their area of service. Just as patients sought to enact moral relations by bringing providers into kinship relations, bureaucrats sought to enact their own understanding of what constituted a moral relation between providers and the wider community they served.

Efforts to provide a systematic warm care through data collection highlighted how state projects to reenvision care remained rooted in liberal mechanisms of governance and accountability. Simultaneously, I suggest, the surveys' approach to social determinants largely continued to locate risk in community members' individual and household practices, as well as in their kin relations. In doing so, they extended the pathologization of Indigenous bodies and relations at the root of colonial care. As scholars of Indigenous data sovereignty have demonstrated, dominant paradigms for data collection often rely on modes of asking questions, framing populations, and measuring processes and outcomes that reflect colonial presuppositions about Indigenous peoples (Kukutai and Taylor 2016; Locklear, Hesketh, Begay, Brixey, Echo-Hawk, and James 2023). Under such rubrics, data measurement and analysis can sidestep the historical and structural roots of health inequality, instead rooting damage within Indigenous populations themselves (see Tuck 2009).[3] As Dian Million puts it, "[L]arge data descriptions of Indigenous anomie eclipse the specifics and sources of our suffering, and perhaps more importantly, our specific strengths, silencing the narratives of the strengths of our actual lives or the conditions of our actual deaths" (2020, 401).

On the day I accompanied GHA staffers to complete the surveys, Mariela took a few minutes to fill out the remainder of the form before moving on to the next house. On the first page, she tabulated Paulino's responses to her questions to assess the risk level of his household.

The form assigned a numerical value to each response. Families who slept with over five people in a single room, for example, were marked twenty-five "risk" points, while those who slept with one to two in a room were only marked five. Burning one's trash amounted to four points, while burying it was worth three. After filling out the survey, health personnel added up the numbers from the responses: 28 to 61 points was a low-risk family, 62 to 126 was medium risk, and 127 to 165 was high risk.

After she had calculated the household's risk level, in one of the blank squares on the first page of the survey, Mariela sketched out a rough map of where Paulino's house was located in the village, so that another practitioner could find it again. In the other blank square, she sketched out a kinship chart (called a *familiograma*) of Paulino's household based on his responses. Providers were expected to sketch family connections using squares, circles, and triangles, resembling the forms of kin mapping that had once been common practice in anthropological fieldwork. In addition to marking blood relations, illnesses, births, and deaths on the kinship chart, health personnel were expected to qualify the relationships between members of the family as "close," "very close," "distant," "conflictive," or "ruptured." For example, a "close" relationship was illustrated with a straight line between family members, while a "conflictive" relationship was drawn with a zigzag line. A "ruptured" relationship showed a break in the straight lines connecting family members (Ministerio de Salud de Bolivia 2014, 235).[4]

Mariela marked Paulino's familial relationships with the simple straight line that stood for "close"—as she did for all other households she visited that day. Following this pattern, in a box on the second page of the form that asked surveyors to evaluate family behavior (*comportamiento familiar*) as either "functional" or "dysfunctional," she checked off Paulino's family as "functional." When I asked Mariela how she assessed whether a family was functional or dysfunctional, she paused, mulling over the question. She suggested dysfunctional families might include those in which the father was absent. In the surveys she filled out that day, she marked the families as "functional" in all but a few instances: a family in which the mother had died, another whose father had abandoned them.

In the context of the Bolivian carpetas, policy efforts to account for wider social conditions and relations were ultimately folded back into a narrower model of individualized health risk. Emily Yates-Doerr reminds us that interventions designed to address the "social determinants of health" come from a progressive desire to move beyond individual blame and attend to the social underpinnings of health inequality. Yet, as she argues, social determinants frameworks often predetermine what constitutes both "the social" and "health," offering "prescriptive solutions that often do not result in the deep structural transformation they claim to inspire" (2020, 380). The carpetas narrowly fixed the conditions shaping health through forms of documenting and seeing that centered on a normative model of the functional family comprising a mother, father, and children. It foregrounded a preoccupation with domestic practices such as food consumption and how many people slept in a room. Kin relations were scripted as potential sources of illness that could be weighted numerically. Replicating long-standing racializing tropes of the Indigenous family as a site of deviance and pathology, surveys marked "the normal" and "the pathological" not only onto health, illness, and the body but also onto the family itself as a site of regulation and concern (see Foucault 1980). As numerous scholars have shown, colonial biopolitics historically took bourgeois intimacy within the private domain of the household as its reference point—and sought to criminalize, regulate, and transform colonized subjects' practices of kinship, sexuality, and domesticity (Kauanui 2018; Lowe 2015; Stoler 1995; 2010). The stickiness and endurance of kinship as a site of pathology and biopolitical intervention foreclosed the more holistic and relational understanding of health to which many policymakers aspired. It also bracketed providers off from the relations constituting patients' well-being. Instead, patient kin relations (understood primarily in terms of biology and the household) became sites of potential pathology in need of monitoring.

Still, while these relations and practices were defined as "risky," their precise implications for health remained indeterminate. Take, for example, the question about how many people slept in a room. Many parents shared rooms with their children; sometimes, the whole family slept in one room. When I asked policymakers and NGO workers why this practice posed a health risk, they were not sure, nor was an explanation detailed in the instructions. I continued to wonder if the question was designed to be a stand-in for measuring household income, or whether sharing a room posed a health risk because of possible contagion between persons. I also could never determine why, on the numerical scale, this practice posed a much greater health risk than burning one's trash.

In practice, the production of data about risk remained contingent on providers' labor, judgment, and discretion. For many providers, the surveys were a burdensome, time-consuming task in addition to the many other tasks they already had to undertake.[5] Hospital and health post practitioners were already stretched thin—and, as with the day I accompanied Mariela, NGO providers sometimes had to step in to ensure the surveys were completed by the deadline. Biomedical providers and the NGO workers who helped them quickly went through the questions on the surveys, using the form's numerical guides to assess risk. When Mariela put "close" and "functional" relations as the default in most cases, she reckoned with what she did not (or could not) know based on a brief survey encounter. If she adhered to survey questions about family structure and household practices, she also used her own judgment and discretion when engaging interlocutors, suggesting that most people she met were not in need of special concern or intervention. As with many forms of data collection, the carpetas created a central paradox: interpersonal negotiations and judgments were essential to producing legible data (Biruk 2018)—even as the technical and coherent appearance of finalized data concealed the very indeterminacy of data collection (Scherz 2011).[6]

After the surveys were completed, the Machacamarca Hospital statistician entered them into a computerized database for the entire municipality. Under the SAFCI policy, each health establishment was also required to create a *sala situacional* (situational room) that displayed maps of community risk levels and charts of health indicators.

For the final project for the SAFCI training course (see Chapter 2), Dr. Lydia had the providers use the data from the files to develop visuals to hang up in the hospital's main meeting room, transforming it into a sala situacional. I joined the hospital providers as they mapped the data by hand-coloring in households on a map for each district (using municipal government maps for the urbanized area of Machacamarca and hand-drawn maps for the more rural areas of the municipality). We spent hours poring over the rough maps drawn on the files of houses (there were no addresses or house numbers) and tried to match them with their counterparts on the official, but outdated, map of Machacamarca. Using pencils, we colored in the households according to their medical risk level from the charts: red for high risk, yellow for medium risk, and green for low risk (Figure 5.1). Another group was charged with tying colored strings on the binding of the family files (likewise in green, yellow, or red) so that the risk level would be easily identifiable if a doctor needed to pull the file off the shelf (Figure 5.2). Circulating in the room as the groups worked, I overheard bursts of laughter and cries of frustration as practitioners attempted to match

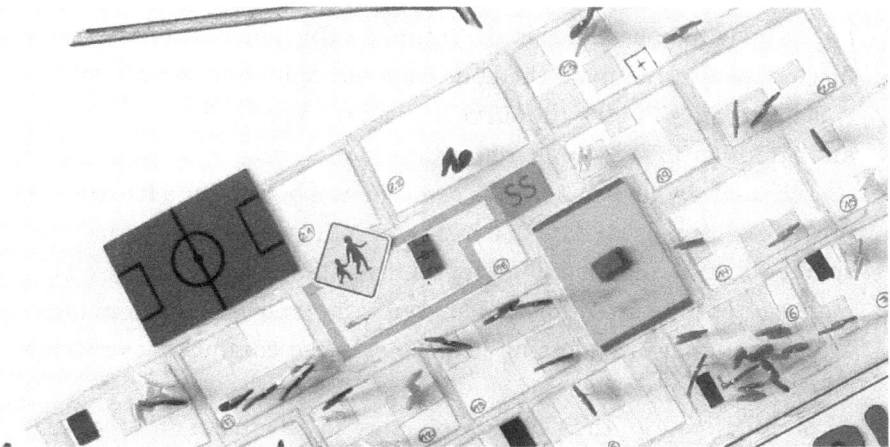

FIGURE 5.1. Part of a painstakingly hand-colored map hung up in the Machacamarca Hospital's *sala situacional*. (Photograph has been edited to remove identifiable street names). Source: Photograph by the author.

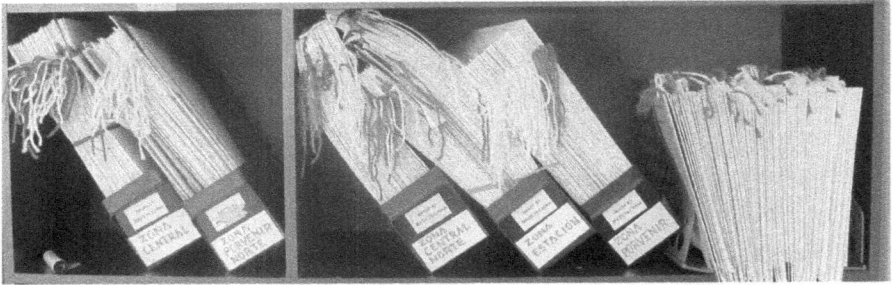

FIGURE 5.2. A shelf in the *sala situacional* of the collected household surveys, organized by neighborhood and color-coded by risk level. Source: Photograph by the author.

the rough hand-drawn maps of houses on the files with the maps provided by the municipality. They joked and gossiped with each other as they worked and called across the room for others to pass them pencils or strings of different colors.

Tasks like coloring in maps and color-coding files with risk levels encouraged providers to care for data sets, even as they also reckoned with the limits of implementation. The purpose of the sala situacional was to aid providers in visualizing the communities they served and follow up with households in the future. In the Bolivian context, state discourses firmly linked the collection of population health data to warm care, positioning the surveys as a new mechanism of inclusion and attention to patients' circumstances. Coloring in maps and cutting colored strings was a tactile, sometimes laborious and frustrating practice of visualizing data that had been collected (albeit one that also sparked humor and laughter). Yet for practitioners, it could also be a means of putting attention and energies into knowing a community, of insisting that providers no longer neglected communities as they had done in the past.

Simultaneously, the creation of salas situacionales in Machacamarca and elsewhere was intended to signal to local residents that health establishments were attending to their concerns. Although the Machacamarca Hospital meeting room was most often used for hospital staff meetings, it was also the site for participatory planning meetings with local community representatives. The sala situacional was visually striking and inviting. With its bright, hand-drawn maps and data visualizations, one might even say that it was playful. It interrupted the austere laboratory-like architecture of the hospital that had long been a symbol of assimilative progress. Presenting collected data in a semi-public, invitingly playful way was a means for practitioners to feel engaged with the community they were serving; it also reminded community representatives that hospital practitioners were tuned into community health problems and actively working to remedy them. Like other projects I have described in this book, it melded bureaucratic technologies with a discursive and affective emphasis on warmth and inclusion.

Yet as the hospital practitioners recounted, no one had, as yet, used the data when treating patients or conducting household checkups. The surveys sat untouched on the shelves of the sala situacional. Providers were supposed to return to visit "red" and "yellow" houses more frequently—but those I interviewed described difficulty finding the time to do so. As with the collection of the initial data, follow-up household visits were challenging to complete alongside their other work responsibilities. In other words, it was difficult to mobilize biomedical practitioners with limited time and resources to conduct follow-up visits. As resource and labor constraints meant that collective surveys often sat on the shelf, the labor of data collection and display itself became the central mode of enacting warm care. Yet, for patients, answering the survey questions did not lead to greater access to health resources or to resource redistribution in their favor.

It was perhaps not surprising, then, that some residents of the municipality reacted skeptically to the survey—by associating it with other forms of state taxation and dispossession (as Delina recounted) or (as I often observed) by showing caution when answering. Like Paulino, many people whose households we visited answered questions in ways that aligned with dominant institutional norms, including by emphasizing their adherence to biomedicine, avoidance of traditional healers, and consumption of healthy foods. In contrast to the healers

I described in Chapter 4, who reappropriated bureaucratic technologies in their efforts to establish exchange relations with institutions, patients rarely engaged more actively with the carpetas in making claims. Carpetas were not administered frequently, nor did they seem to be connected to material outcomes. On the day I accompanied Mariela, a few people asked if answering the survey would mean that the doctor would come treat them for medical problems—and Mariela always responded that while it would not lead to direct care, the data collection would help providers understand health issues "to better the health of the community."

DOCTORS, ANTHROPOLOGISTS, AND ACCOUNTABILITY ACROSS HIERARCHIES

What might it mean, then, to imagine kinship differently? To understand kinship not as a site of scrutiny and risk, but as a way of tying practitioners and patients together—of imbricating them in each other's lives? How might such relations reshape the terms of care, with effects on the body, health, and well-being?

Despite the Ministry of Health's nominal embrace of Indigenous relationality as a paradigm of care, the surveys' framing of social relations ultimately displaced patients' own understandings of how relations came to bear on health and healing. Even so, while Delina and others worried the carpetas were making it more difficult to gain patients' trust, many residents of the municipality continued to bring biomedical practitioners—as well as anthropologists like me—into kin relations.

On a rare rainy day in 2015, I accompanied my neighbor Augusto and his grandson, Javi, to the hospital. Javi was a slight, six-year-old boy who often wore a furry fleece hat in the shape of a tiger slung over his large ears. Augusto, worried that his usually energetic grandson had become pale, tired, and without appetite, had decided to take him to see a doctor.

Javi's father had died some time ago, and his mother had left to work as a seamstress in Argentina for several years. His extended family was taking care of him until his mother returned. Augusto thought I might especially be of use when he took Javi to the hospital. I had already been conducting ethnographic research in the hospital for several months, and I knew most of the staff there. Augusto reasoned that if I came along, Javi would be certain to receive better care.

Augusto's intuitions were not far off. We arrived early in the morning to get an appointment slip and lined up in the hallway for several hours outside the already bursting waiting room. When the nurse finally called out Javi's name and motioned us to come through, the practitioners were friendly and attentive. They said that, of course, they would do everything they could to help my friends.

We spent the day in the hospital, shuttling between the pediatrician, the X-ray technician, and finally the telemedicine room. There, a general medical practitioner used a shiny computer—easily the newest piece of equipment in the hospital—to place a video call to a pulmonologist in the capital city of La Paz. She held up the worrisome X ray the technician had taken of Javi's chest, which showed a rib cage engulfed in a bright white mass. On the screen, the pulmonologist squinted at the image and proclaimed, "It might be a parasite. Or an abscess. Or it might be cancer. Tell the family to bring the patient to La Paz so I can run tests." Augusto, sitting in the corner, glanced at me worriedly. La Paz was several hours away, and the family did not know anyone there who could host them. Javi, moreover, did not have insurance.[7]

As we were about to leave, I went to thank the doctors and found them huddling in the hallway, still looking at the X ray. "It's probably a parasite," they insisted. "But we can't be sure." They suggested I snap a photo of the X ray on my phone to show the rest of the family, so that I could explain to them the urgency of going to La Paz.

When we returned home, I spoke to Pablo, who was Augusto's son and Javi's uncle. He had traveled to the city that morning to buy animal feed and was unloading the heavy, blue tarp bags from the back of his car. Hesitating over how to explain Javi's diagnosis—or lack thereof—I spotted Dr. Mauricio, one of the hospital's general practitioners, walking on the side of the road and waved him over. He had not been at the hospital that morning, but he was a good friend of the family and their compadre. Pablo lamented to the doctor that Javi was sick, and

I showed both of them the blurry photo of the X ray on my knock-off Samsung. We stood in a circle around that small image that appeared to hold a hidden truth about Javi's condition that no one could quite grasp.

Pablo choked. "If it's cancer, it's better that he stay home to die with his family."

Dr. Mauricio tried to reassure him. "Looking at this, I would say that it's probably just a parasite. They can operate on that in La Paz. He will be fine."

Javi ultimately did have a cyst caused by a parasite and was able to obtain treatment at a hospital in La Paz—although his challenging journey to obtain care in the city is not one that I recount here. Instead, I draw attention to the relations that unfolded at this early stage. As the family sought a diagnosis, Dr. Mauricio and I were brought into relations of social and ethical obligation. Dr. Mauricio was Pablo's compadre of several years, and as such, he was a trusted source of information. I, in turn, lived with members of Javi's extended family but was also a researcher working in the hospital; as such, I also became a resource for accessing care. Some months after these events transpired—and Javi had the surgery to remove the parasite in La Paz—I was asked to become a godmother to his younger sister.

In writing about kinship, it is impossible to separate out my participation in these practices. Just as patients urged providers to not separate themselves from the social relations that constituted health, many of my neighbors urged me to understand myself as part of a densely woven network of ethical obligations. Living and working in Machacamarca, I came to know many of my neighbors well. Often read as a gringa—as someone with relatively greater wealth and a foreign passport—I was asked to become a godmother numerous times over the course of my research, in addition to participating in other forms of exchanging gifts and favors.

Max Liboiron, in conversation with Shawn Wilson (2008), argues that accountability is a key mode of relating to others that should also guide research ethics. Their understanding of accountability is distinct from the kinds of bureaucratic accountability built into data collection, which mobilized surveys to cultivate systematic care. Instead, Liboiron emphasizes that in many Indigenous communities "fulfilling a role and obligations" is a way to be "accountable to your relations" (2021, 121). In Machacamarca, kinship and exchange practices enacted long-term, sometimes laborious, forms of mutual accountability across social hierarchies. As a researcher working in the area, I was expected to fulfill a role and obligations in multiple ways: to accompany patients during medical visits, to become a godmother, to provide gifts of food (in exchange for other gifts of food), to share research findings, to continue visiting even after I had left Machacamarca and my research was over. Such practices also shaped how I came to be in relation with others, both within and outside the context of research. Yet while I consider several people I worked with to be kin (and they consider me their kin as well), that never erased my position as gringa, settler, or researcher; it simply shaped the terms of obligation. As Alison Jones and Kuni Jenkins (2008) argue, claims to mutuality can be mobilized by researchers as a form of erasing or sidestepping the entrenched realities of power. Practices of obligation were never about pretending a hierarchy did not exist, but about creating forms of accountability across that hierarchy.

As I worked to build accountable relations, I also reflected on the roles biomedical practitioners were expected to play when they were brought into exchanges or asked to be godparents. Bringing biomedical practitioners into relationships of kinship and exchange likewise did not entail shedding hierarchies; instead, they sought to facilitate morally appropriate enactments of authority (Leinaweaver 2008; Winchell 2022; Van Vleet 2008). Habituated forms of care practice could work to maintain existing social orders (Aulino 2019), while also reconfiguring them to create an ethical ground for accountability, solidarity, and intimacy (Scherz 2014).

In Machacamarca, people did not make a one-to-one calculus that asking a biomedical provider (or an anthropologist) to become kin was a means to gain access to medical care in the moment. Instead, they expected that, as part of relations of obligation, people would enact moral duties as they emerged. Dr. Mauricio was not present at the hospital that day, but because he was obliged to the family, he was willing to help them decipher the X ray and discuss next steps. While I had been asked to accompany Javi and Augusto, I did not get asked to be a godmother to Javi's younger sister until much later, after Javi was already better, and when I had already proven that I was reliably in relation with the family.

For hospital staff to be asked to be godparents, they already had to exhibit good qualities—to be the kind of person one might want to be kin. Such judgments—about who was a good practitioner and who was not—bridged multiple moral expectations. Practitioners had to show attentiveness and generosity, but also have a certain social status. In the Machacamarca Hospital, patients mostly asked doctors—and especially male doctors—to become godparents. There were some exceptions: a few had close relationships with nurses, like Adriana, who had lived and worked in the town for over a decade. It was usually the doctor, however, who became the renowned figure that people sought.

In Machacamarca, people often recounted that Dr. Mauricio was one of the best doctors at the hospital. A gregarious general medical practitioner from the eastern lowlands of Santa Cruz, he spoke quickly, lopping off the s's at the ends of words, and joked frequently with patients. Sometimes, he attempted a few words in Aymara—textbook words pertaining to health and illness, as well as risqué jokes that people had taught him over the course of his years working in the small town. Unlike many practitioners I came to know who transferred out of Machacamarca after a few years when they could find a job in the city, Dr. Mauricio had been there for over a decade.

When I accompanied Dr. Mauricio during his shifts at the hospital, he took a long time attending to each of his patients. In between shifts, he would sometimes take phone calls from prior patients or attend to them outside his regular clinic hours. Other hospital workers expressed their frustrations because he took too long when seeing patients and was easily distracted. Yet many patients sought him out as a person who might grant them attentiveness in an otherwise unstable medical context.

According to what people told me, Dr. Mauricio was one of the few general medical practitioners they considered *de confianza* (trust-worthy)—which set him apart from many other practitioners working at their local institution. Some years ago, there had been more doctors who were de confianza working in the hospital. My neighbor Hector rang their names off for me like a well-rehearsed list: Dr. Mauricio, Dr. Jaime, Dr. Wilson, and Dr. Elena. He lamented that the municipal government had not paid these doctors enough, prompting them to leave for better jobs in the cities of La Paz and El Alto. Even now, people recalled them with nostalgic affection, recounting how such-and-such was *un buen doctor*—a good doctor. Most practitioners who were asked to become kin agreed to do so. Often, they were asked when they had already come to know patients fairly well—and it was also another means for them to gain respect in a community. Dr. Mauricio, for example, frequently spoke of the many *ahijados* (godchildren) he had in and around Machacamarca.

Yet this practice also sometimes encountered limits as a site of transforming medical care. Kin-work could be onerous and required continual presence and following up on obligations. It could entail, for example, showing up for celebrations, paying for gifts, continually contributing time and labor in the long term. When I returned to Machacamarca to visit in 2019, Javi's parents, who had returned to Machacamarca after several years of working in a factory in Argentina, were furious. A few years after Dr. Mauricio had helped with Javi's care, they had asked the doctor to become godfather to their younger son. Yet on the day of the baptism, he had failed to show up. Busy with work, the doctor had forgotten.

REDEFINING HEALTH

While such modes of kinship were laborious and could sometimes fall through, they became a central terrain not just for shaping the terms of care but also for sustaining health itself. In 2015, I sat down for an interview with my neighbor Rosa, an Aymara woman in her late thirties. Sixteen years prior to our conversation, her infant son had lost his soul when she took him down to the river. A child's soul did not become firmly entrenched until adolescence, and incidents that sparked fright or sorrow could easily cause the soul to flee (Canessa 2012; Crandon-Malamud 1991). In those days, Rosa still lived in her home village, some distance from Machacamarca. She took her baby with her as she went to wash clothes and bathe in the stream that carved a narrow path through tufts of yellowed grass. Some women she did not know offered to hold him—and because of that, he fell ill.

At the time, she was sure he would die. She tried desperately to breastfeed him, but he would not accept any milk because of his fright. Yet as she was caring for her baby, she spotted Lucy, a young doctor who sometimes came to the village to vaccinate its inhabitants and treat the sick. Rosa, recounting the story many years later, told me,

> Lucy is my comadre. She used to work in those times in the hospital. She came to visit the community. She always came, but she happened to show up at that moment. So, she told me, "Baptize your son. If not, he will die. But this way, he will live." This is what she said. "Ok," I said. "But who will go [find the priest]?" "I have my car. I will go," she said, and she came. She brought the priest to my father-in-law's house, and he baptized [my son]. My son was not baptized in the Church. . . . So, Lucy was now my comadre. She was a doctor. She was very young. . . . Afterwards I got [my son] cured. I had his soul called. He healed.

Hesitating over her words, I asked, "Was Lucy the one who cured him?"

Rosa shook her head. "No, it was another person."

"A *curandero* [healer]?" I asked.

Rosa nodded. "Yes, a healer called back his soul. Yes. With that he was better."

In our conversation, my first instinct was to piece together a clear linearity of events and determine whether Lucy had made any efforts to treat the infant, as I assumed a doctor would. Yet for Rosa, the doctor was not the central figure who had cured her son. Rather, Lucy was one of several people who facilitated the process of healing. If Rosa's son had lost his soul when being held by strangers, his soul was returned with the help of multiple persons: the doctor who prompted the baptism and became kin in the process, the priest who would safeguard the soul through baptism, the healer who would call the soul to return.

Rosa and Lucy also shared a lasting bond, which opened up other possibilities for care in the future. Many years later, Rosa's relative was transferred to a hospital in La Paz, where Lucy had gone on to work after leaving her post in the countryside. Rosa called her to find out if she still had contacts in the hospital who could help move up the surgery.

Just as cultivating the right forms of care could heal the effects of alienation (see Chapter 4), participating in these relations of long-term kinship and obligation with doctors could also sustain bodily wellness. Medical anthropologists have long shown how gifting exchange practices—such as gifts of food (Street 2014) or providing envelopes of money to doctors (Praspaliauskiene 2016)—can both facilitate care and transform the body itself. In contrast to a biomedical and public health focus on monitoring kinship practices, many patients understood biomedicine to function effectively when it was folded into kin relations. Rosa and Lucy's relationship centered on a long-term sense of mutual obligation—favors that could be called in over many years in and out of the confines of the hospital. It also exceeded any fixed categorization of "traditional" versus "modern" medicine. Initially, Lucy ceded her place to the priest and then to the healer. Yet years later, when Rosa's family member was sick, she also facilitated his access to biomedical care in the hospital. Care, in this instance, was not the immediate interaction of diagnosis and cure, but a longer commitment that could be deferred and taken up when needed.

In Machacamarca, providers who engaged in appropriate relations, who properly enacted their authority, were also often assumed to be potent healers. Pablo, for example, insisted that his compadre Dr. Victor had "hands that could cure." He described it to me later: merely being examined by the doctor, who had the touch, was enough to make him healthier. Yet not all doctors had this ability. Rather, it was usually someone with whom one had a close relation who had the ability to heal and transfer a sense of wellness to their patient. This did not replace medications or other components of biomedical treatment—which still came afterwards—but it had a profound bodily effect different from the feeling of "no care."

———

Toward the end of my stay in Machacamarca, I sat down for an interview with Dr. Wilmer, the director of the hospital. We had chatted informally many times before then, crossing paths in meetings and workshops held for the biomedical practitioners in the hospital. During our conversation, he expressed his concern that some patients were trying to take advantage:

> We are always telling [health care providers] that in this hospital we provide care that, in some form, respects everyone as equals. So, we are trying to make it so that it's not like before, when the doctor, or the health personnel, was above the patient. Now, we are trying to balance it, make it horizontal. But in some form also making sure health personnel are respected. Because there are many people, with the government of Evo Morales and all that, who exaggerate. Sometimes, they think that because they are part of the government, because they are Indigenous, they have a right to everything. And that's not true. There needs to be equilibrium, between respect for them and for us. And so, we also try to take care of that aspect, because there is everything. There are excesses on the side of the people, and there are also some excesses on the side of the doctors. So, we are trying to create an equilibrium so that everything is horizontal.

As others working in Bolivia have noted, institutional actors have often mobilized liberal frameworks against practices of patronage and compadrazgo, couching these as antithetical to ideals of individual autonomy and equality (Ellison 2018; Winchell 2022). Under Evo Morales, state officials also centrally embraced an understanding of liberation that hinged on individual rights and freedoms, rendering local Indigenous practices of kinship and exchange problematic for the state (Winchell 2022). Echoing the provider narratives I described in Chapter 2, Dr. Wilmer emphasized that biomedical practitioners were committed to a new politics of equality for all. In his view, it was patients who were disrupting that politics of equality—who were engaging in excess, who expected too much.[8]

While many practitioners did ultimately agree to become kin, Dr. Wilmer's doubts highlighted the centrality of liberal discourses of equality to biomedical care and the tensions that emerged around questions of kinship and exchange. New technologies like the household survey were in line with ideals of bureaucratic consistency, equality, and making patients knowable to both local health establishments and the state. In moving away from the uneven contingencies of the interpersonal relation, the surveys rendered kinship as a site of biopolitical surveillance and intervention, rather than a dynamic that providers were also a part of. Yet these bureaucratic transformations also had complex effects. For Delina, building personal relations was essential to community health work—and bureaucratization could bring new challenges to building trust. Care instead was routed in new ways, as practitioners came to attend to and visualize community data sets. Yet for patients, the surveys also did little to bring material changes—as data collection did not necessarily translate into services or greater attention from biomedical practitioners.

As I have described throughout this chapter, patient kin relations were central to rerouting conditions of care. State benevolence has long been intimately tied to racializing projects of improvement; exchange-based moral practices and expectations became a means of rendering that benevolence differently, into forms that were both more moral and more livable for patients. Kin relations with providers required work, and they could also be fraught and burdensome. But they emerged as important sites of meaning that challenged the scope of how the carpetas framed health, as well as the project of warm care more broadly.

6 ACCOUNTABLE CARE

Participatory Planning and the Practice of Complaint

ON A COLD MORNING IN 2015, I sat in the waiting room of the Machaca-marca Hospital. The room was packed with people waiting long hours for their name to be called: the elderly sitting where they could rest their feet, women carrying babies strapped in bright pink fabrics across their backs, small children playing tag and skidding across the dusty tile floor. I spotted my neighbor Hector sitting against the far wall, and he gestured at me to join him, glad for some company to pass the time.

Hector was a middle-aged Aymara man who, whenever we encoun-tered one another, frequently turned to describing his frustrations with national politics. That morning, he turned his ire to the dete-riorating clinical infrastructure that surrounded us. He described to me how "Evo"—the familiar name almost everyone in Machacamarca used to refer to the president—had promised that life would change. Years before he became president, Evo had spent the night in Mach-acamarca as he led protestors down the highway on a march to the capital city. "Evo said he would repay us for our hospitality. But now he has forgotten us," Hector insisted. He rang off a list of unfulfilled promises. The hospital was still falling apart, and there was no care.

Moreover, the construction of the promised new stadium down the road was never completed. And so on and so forth.

In Bolivian Spanish, the verb *renegar* means to complain or grumble, often in a ranting fashion. It also becomes a noun to describe someone who makes a habit of complaining: *renegón* (m.) and *renegona* (f.).[1] To renegar—especially about politics—was a common mode and affect of speech, in Machacamarca and elsewhere in Bolivia. Yet it was also, I suggest in this chapter, a generative site of political engagement. In Machacamarca, where many residents had voted for Evo Morales and the MAS, *renegando* (complaining) also became a site for articulating obligations and demands for accountability in the aftermath of activism.

Practices of renegando unfolded across many formal and informal sites. Although I also bring in offhand conversations—like the one with Hector—in this chapter, I primarily focus on complaint as it unfolded in spaces created for grassroots participation in health planning at the local level. While neoliberal reformers first enacted popular participation policies in the 1990s (Cameron 2009a; 2009b; Postero 2007), the Morales administration repositioned participatory health planning as part of a more progressive agenda: local participation would grant a central decision-making role to social movements and contribute to decolonizing the national health care system. One goal of decolonizing health care was to bring representatives from grassroots organizations—unions, ayllus, and neighborhood associations that were central to local communal governance—into the process of municipal health planning. To facilitate participation, the SAFCI policy proposed the creation of "spaces of deliberation" (*espacios de deliberación*)—including municipal assemblies, roundtables, and committee meetings—where grassroots representatives could meet with health personnel to discuss health problems in the community and put forward proposals to include in the yearly municipal health plan. Participatory health planning also required the formation of a local health committee, made up of local grassroots organization members, who would take the lead in articulating local health needs. Like many other initiatives I have described in this book, while the meetings were required by national law, they were often supported and facilitated by GHA staffers, who provided food and equipment and sometimes stepped in to explain key tenets of national policy and how to put forward proposals. I dwell on these "spaces of deliberation" because they were central sites where complaints came to the fore, revealing both possibilities and tensions within the state project.

For many people who complained during these participatory health planning meetings, the Morales administration had fallen short of its promises of transformation. Many of them had participated in the social movements against neoliberal privatization that had brought Evo Morales to the presidency; many of them also continued to vote for Evo Morales and the MAS. Simultaneously, they worried out loud about the limitations of what his administration had been able to accomplish. In the context of health care, planning-meeting participants frequently couched demands for greater transformation in terms of complaints about what was not working. Complaints frequently focused on a dearth of basic health infrastructure and on problems of practitioner mistreatment in clinical settings. Both were issues that Ministry of Health officials had promised to address. In bringing these complaints into participatory planning spaces, participants publicly disrupted state narratives that the Morales administration (in contrast to prior administrations) was providing for poor and Indigenous patients. Complaint, I argue, was less a wholesale rejection of his administration's policies and approaches than a demand that it keep to its promises.

In this context, state officials interpreted complaint as both an expected and an unruly practice. It was expected in the sense that officials foregrounded the centrality of grassroots organizations to the Morales administration's governing strategy and understood pushback to be a central form of political engagement. But it was also unruly in the sense that institutional actors perceived complainers to not know how to make demands for health correctly—and to be pushing back unnecessarily against institutional offers of care. To this end, officials running meetings frequently sought to tamp down, redirect, or, as Susan Ellison (2018) puts it, "domesticate" unruly complaints. As officials struggled to implement promised policies under constrained resources, they sought to reroute complaints in ways that maintained the narrative of a state that cared.

As Sara Ahmed writes, "You can become a complainer because of where you locate the problem. To become a complainer is to become the location of a problem" (2021, 3). But by "giving complaint a hearing" (3), we might also engage a key record of frustration and confrontation that "[teaches] us something about how institutions work" (6). With this in mind, I ask what possibilities participants opened up by engaging in complaint. Moving away from the idea that complaint is an inherently negative or unproductive practice, I demonstrate how complaint laid the groundwork for institutional accountability. Sitting with the comments of Hector and others, I understand complaint to be a politically important and generative site for pushing against the limits of state reform—and the limits of warm care. It opened up possibilities for participants to generatively rework—and sometimes rupture—their relationships with state and development agencies.

ACTIVISM AND ITS AFTERMATHS

In the tumultuous years preceding Evo Morales's election to the presidency in 2005, the Gas War in the cities of El Alto and La Paz reverberated in the much smaller town of Machacamarca. The protests were sparked when the neoliberal president Gonzalo Sánchez de Lozada proposed to export Bolivia's natural gas supplies via a pipeline through Chile. But protesters also connected the pipeline to wider and long-standing concerns about neoliberal structural adjustment, privatization, and wealth inequality (Bjork-James 2020; Gustafson 2020). As many residents of Machacamarca later told me, they joined the national protests by blockading the highway that ran through town and all the way to the twin cities of El Alto and La Paz. Because of its location on a major national roadway, Machacamarca had frequently been a strategic point for protestors to halt traffic by rolling tires into the road. In the town and surrounding villages, members of the local branches of the CSUTCB, Bolivia's largest national peasant union, also traveled up to the city of El Alto to join the larger protests.

It was a memory that many Machacamarqueños carried with them when they described what the state under Evo Morales owed them. During a community health meeting in a village near Machacamarca, a union leader named Ricardo stood up to complain that he had given his blood for Evo but had gotten nothing in return. His village's health post was still missing medications, and the ambulances they were promised never arrived. The language of complaint frequently invoked in public forums reflected a desire to call upon the president—and the state—to remember its obligations.

The history of the Gas War and other major protests during Bolivia's two decades of neoliberalism show how Evo Morales and the MAS emerged out of a series of complaints—although the genre of the complaint (via speech-making, protests, and other demands of the state) also had a much longer history in Bolivia. This was a history that the Morales administration also leaned into by promising to make social movement participation a centerpiece of its politics (Anria 2018; McNelly 2023). As Thomas Grisaffi notes in his study on Bolivian coca grower unions, Morales vocally promised to "lead by obeying," inviting "the rank and file to treat him as if he were nothing more than another union member, using phrases such as 'tell me when I make a mistake,' 'please guide me,' 'this is not the government of Evo Morales alone, this is our government'" (2019, 6).

Yet in public forums such as spaces of community participation, local representatives were now engaging in complaint to demand accountability from the MAS. Although the population of the Machacamarca municipality tended to vote overwhelmingly for the MAS for the presidential elections (less so for regional and local elections), they also expressed a range of perspectives on both the possibilities and the limits of state reform during Evo Morales's administration. For many, Morales's presidency had led to rising standards of living and a more representative state—but these key transformations had also failed to translate into improved conditions of health care. In this context, complaining—in private or in public—became a means of reflecting on and making demands for the fulfillment of state obligations.

But complaints were also predicated, in part, on the hope that state officials would engage and listen because of the MAS's stated commitment to social movements. This held true even for community members who were not MAS voters. I came to better understand this dynamic when I spoke to Emilia, a middle-aged member of the municipal governing council who had been put in charge of local health projects. The new municipal government had just been elected, representing the Patriotic Socialist Alliance, one of several new, small, left-wing parties that had edged out the once-dominant MAS in Bolivian regional elections. Emilia explained to me that one of the party's main goals was to expand the hospital and transform it into the second-tier regional center that had initially been promised to the municipality. The sticking point, however, was the funding—which the municipal government could never afford on its own.

Emilia told me that her plan was to arrange a meeting with President Morales and ask him to fund it. I knew from my research that the construction of health infrastructures usually required petitioning the Departmental Health Service and the Ministry of Health—yet the bureaucratic process was long, onerous, and unlikely to bring results. I also wondered whether a local councilwoman would be able to obtain a meeting with the president himself. Yet her efforts to obtain a meeting with the president as the most feasible solution for expanding the hospital pointed to what was still a personalized relationship with a state that could also follow up on promises and obligations.

Emilia's moral expectations reflected her hope that the state might fulfill its promises of transforming health care and acting on behalf of Indigenous, poor, and working-class Bolivians. If Machacamarqueños frequently expected the state to hold to its obligations of redistribution (see Chapter 4), they especially hoped that the MAS's own social movement history might make it receptive to hearing demands. Such expectations, in other words, were bound up with the idea that the state, despite its shortcomings, might still listen. However, as I describe further on, state and NGO officials also worked to reroute these claims into forms that they deemed to be more feasible and productive.

WAYS OF TALKING ABOUT HEALTH

One day, I accompanied a small group of three GHA staffers to the main meeting hall in the village of R, not far from Machacamarca, for a municipal health planning meeting. As required by national law, Dr. Wilmer, the Machacamarca Hospital director (who also served as director of health programs for the municipality) was supposed to meet periodically with select staff from the hospital and surrounding health posts, members of the municipal government and local health committee, and local civil society representatives. In Machacamarca, the category of civil society members encompassed the two main peasant syndicates in the region—known as the "Túpac Kataris" for the men and the "Bartolina Sisas" for the women[2]—as well as members of neighborhood associations (*juntas vecinales*) from the urbanized area. The location for the meeting always rotated between the four sites in the municipality that housed health establishments. In the chilly meeting hall that day, rural syndicate members—the Bartolina Sisas wearing dark green skirts and the Túpac Kataris wearing dark jackets and fedoras—crowded onto narrow benches. At the front of the room, the syndicate leaders shared a table with the hospital director and a few other biomedical practitioners in front of presentation slides projected directly onto the wall. GHA staffers stood along the walls, circulating to hand out food and writing supplies, occasionally taking photographs for their webpage to document their work in supporting community participation.

After morning introductions and deliberations, we paused to eat lunch—chicken, potatoes, and pasta supplied by GHA. As people wrapped up their meals, Elena, one of the NGO workers, opened a new set of PowerPoint slides and took her place in front of the crowd. Gesturing toward the presentation projected behind her, she asked the group, "Who here knows what the SAFCI is?"

Silence. Elena paused uncertainly for a few seconds, then launched into a broad sketch of the policy's key components, including its emphasis on community participation. "Thanks to our hermano, Evo, you are now in a position to decide," she told her audience.

Writing about the circulation of the SAFCI policy in Bolivia, Alissa Bernstein (2018) highlights how health policy traveled and took shape through various workshop events; didactic sessions were an opportunity both to explain policy and to engage with civil society actors for input. Similarly, I found that many state and NGO actors emphasized the importance of foregrounding local perspectives and challenging top-down approaches, understanding their didactic explanations of the SAFCI policy to further empower community members to participate in local health policy. At the same time, where my findings differ is that many institutional actors also worried out loud that participation was not unfolding in the way they hoped. As Elena later explained to me after the meeting, "Some communities will just hire an accountant to write the municipal health plan. But it doesn't end up representing their needs."

State policymakers I interviewed likewise expressed concerns that opportunities designed for community participation were not productive and that social movement participants did not always know how to make proposals around health care. Fabiola, a bureaucrat at the Ministry of Health, put it this way: "In reality, people don't understand. Or rather, they don't understand what health is." She described needing to mobilize doctors to teach people what health was, especially in the early phases of the SAFCI. Ramón echoed his colleague's sentiments, but blamed people's seeming inability to make the right kinds of demands when it came to health care on the prior colonial state:

> The system has an asistentialista vision, and the population has it even worse. What do they want? They want their hospital, they want one that is third-tier, they want a doctor, they want a CAT scan machine, they want that. This is the first impression of health, and it's because of the focus on treatment that the previous colonial state had. So when you ask them, "Do you want to talk about health?," they associate this with infrastructure, with human resources. But little by little they start to realize. Our concept, our definition of health is more integral, and also has to do with water, with basic conditions, with all these things.

As we continued the conversation, he added, "What we do is facilitate their demand—but not a disordered demand, or one without a head. Rather, it should be an ordered demand. What we try to do is make it so that the organizations have an effective demand, which is systematically presented, which is coherent, which is not too unrealistic, so that they can negotiate with different actors."

In their position as a nonprofit organization facilitating the implementation of national policies at the local level, GHA adopted various strategies for drafting a participatory municipal health plan that, in their view, would better represent community needs. During community planning meetings, they both explained the goals of national health policy and showed PowerPoint slides with health statistics for the community, including rates of illness (for example, for tuberculosis and other endemic problems) and rates of vaccination. GHA staffers also asked health care practitioners to report on the data they had collected from the carpetas familiares and vaccination campaigns—or, if such data was unavailable, to speak about health problems they had observed in person. As I described in Chapter 5, data collection mechanisms like the carpetas familiares revolved around predetermined notions of what constituted a potential health risk; echoing these patterns, the goal was to lay out for participants what constituted health problems in a community that needed addressing. While biomedical practitioners, NGO staffers, and state officials all noted that data collection was often tenuous and there were gaps in knowledge, data nonetheless worked to legitimize what institutional actors considered to be real health problems and interventions.

Critical development studies have highlighted how policies that emphasize the local, the participatory, and the bottom-up, while premised on rectifying the problems of top-down modernization schemes (Scott 1998), can also reentrench relations of power (Cooke and Kothari 2001; Li 2007; Mosse 2005). Scholars have urged us to pay attention to multiple "grammars of participation" (Kelty 2017) as well as the multiple kinds of relations, practices, and interventions they engender. Practices of participatory development, as Ramah McKay puts it, "not only represent but also create local social worlds by constituting and

arraying people, places, and things in ways amenable to nongovern-
mental action" (2018, 45). In Bolivia, emphasis on responsible self-
government had also long been a hallmark of participatory planning
policies since they had been instated under the neoliberal state of the
early 1990s. As Nancy Postero (2007) demonstrates in her study of the
1994 Law of Popular Participation (LPP), NGOs worked closely with
civil society associations to teach them about leadership, rational
language, and other "techniques of the self" they could use to make
claims. Likewise, for John Cameron, the LPP had varied effects: it
provided new mechanisms for Indigenous and peasant groups to gain
control over municipal administrative and development projects, even
as it also risked bureaucratizing and co-opting these struggles (2009b).

The Morales administration emphasized that it was deepening
many of these policies with the goal of building a state oriented around
social movement demands. But as with these earlier iterations of participatory planning, institutional actors leading the discussion also
sought to inculcate specific modes of making demands. Later, during
the same municipal health planning meeting in the village of R, Elena
facilitated a discussion of the issues local peasant leaders wanted addressed when it came to health care. Several representatives for the
Túpac Kataris suggested repairs to their local health post and a more
stable salary line from municipal funds for the sole nurse who staffed
the post. Elena listened and nodded, taking down their points. Then
she said, "Yes, this is all very good. But health is not just infrastructure;
it's also prevention." She proposed several additional interventions to
include in the municipal health plan: education programs for pregnant mothers, drug users, and teenagers; workshops with traditional
healers; empowerment for women leaders. The list presented a com-
pilation of state and NGO priorities, bolstered by local data collection.

Elena's redirecting echoed some of Ramón's concerns that participatory demands were too focused on infrastructure and an asis-
tencialista model of care. Requests for material and infrastructural
investments were common in participatory spaces, even before Morales took office. John Cameron (2009a), in his study of rural Andean
participatory budgeting in the neoliberal era, noted the heavy empha-

sis on requesting projects that required bags of cement. He raised several possibilities that might explain the emphasis on cement-based projects, ranging from the circulation of ideas about modernity and development to the creation of construction jobs, especially given the difficulty finding streams of income in rural areas. As I showed in Chapter 1, under Evo Morales, state officials themselves were also increasingly investing in and publicizing material infrastructure projects like new hospitals. While health policymakers often disagreed on the use of these funds—with some arguing that they needed to be spent instead on primary and preventative care—broader state discourse had also increasingly emphasized material investments as a key marker of state care.

That people might see infrastructural demands as key to transforming care, then, was not surprising. Material investments, as I showed in Chapter 4, were also often markers of the state's willingness to engage in ethics of redistribution and long-term fulfillment of obligations. Given this, many Machacamarqueños understood a lack of care in hospitals and clinics to in part be a problem of resources—and of the state not fulfilling its promises. Simultaneously, some residents of Machacamarca also expressed uncertainty that a better facility might transform the conditions of "no care" in the hospital. That is, gifts of material development aligned in part with projects of modernity, but they did not necessarily rectify the problems of institutional neglect and mistreatment. For example, my neighbor Timoteo argued that the state should invest more in material infrastructures, that Machacamarca was lagging far behind. At the same time, he insisted, he much preferred to treat his stomach ulcers at home, in the care of his family, because doctors were not always very knowledgeable. Rather than seeing such statements as contradictory, I suggest they highlight how multiple aspirations and notions of what might constitute good care were enmeshed. In other words, desires for the state to show care through material investments might coexist with enduring hesitations about the efficacy of biomedical care.

Yet as health infrastructure had been choked through decades of underfunding, state and NGO officials often could not provide consistent streams of equipment and supplies, or funding for new clinics—despite narratives of new state-funded hospitals being built in the cities. Officials sought to direct community members to make demands they deemed both more realistic and more in line with the SAFCI's goals of primary and preventative care.

THE EXPECTED AND THE UNRULY

Amid state and NGO actors' insistence that community members did not know how to talk about health, moments of contention arose frequently during meetings. Although many complaints were about lack of infrastructure, they also sometimes involved extended discussions about mistreatment.

In 2013, I attended a gender and health workshop held by the Ministry of Health in a village called X. X was served by only a small health center, but like the hospital in Machacamarca, it had been fitted with a culturally adapted birthing room, courtesy of GHA. Dr. Carmen, a representative from the Ministry of Health, had traveled from La Paz to talk about women's rights in health in the context of the Morales administration's health reforms with the local branch of the Bartolinas. In this particular case, the ministry's goal was to inform women of their "rights and responsibilities" so that they could better participate in local health care planning.

Women wearing the dark green skirts and pink *aguayos* (cloth wraps) that signaled membership in the agricultural union sat along benches in the dusty and sunlit meeting hall as Dr. Carmen explained the state's new health policies. A mestiza doctor wearing a formal button-down shirt and dark pants, she described how the Morales administration was working to expand access to care and address prior forms of exclusion and discrimination.

Yet as she was speaking, an elderly union member named Victoria interrupted her: "But often, in the hospital, *no hay atención*. That is why we don't go. Our children tend to go more to the health centers. But we are used to curing ourselves with our herbs."

Carmen was momentarily taken aback, pausing in her speech. But she quickly collected herself and responded, "But for some problems it is important to go to the health center. For example, for cervical cancer, nine women die from it every two days in Bolivia. That is to say, 4.5 women die every day."

Dionisia, an older woman sitting near Victoria, chimed in, "But one can get sick from going to the doctor, from the equipment in the health center."

The conversation turned to a rapid, back-and-forth volley:

Carmen: Well, there are some beliefs that aren't true.

Dionisia [*insistent*]: I tell you that I had a friend who got very sick from going to the doctor. Here, we say that the kharikhari [monster that steals the fat from one's body] extracts. But really, it's the doctor who extracts. That's why we don't want to go.

Carmen [*flustered*]: It's true that there are doctors who do their jobs badly. But not all of them are like that.

Victoria: They made my friend do a Cesarian, but she didn't want to. We just prepare our teas, that is all.

Carmen: That is why we have interculturality. Here for example, we have a culturally adapted birthing room. Doctors have realized that the current form of care is not good. They are already working on it. Unfortunately there are some bad experiences, but people can also die if they don't go to the doctor.

Dionisia: But we, too, have our ways of shifting the baby if it's badly positioned. We don't need to go to the doctor.

Carmen: And that's why we also have this process of community participation. One has to dialogue with the health center. One can't just distance oneself.

Victoria: I suppose we have to learn this.

Carmen: We want to eliminate social exclusion, including along lines of gender. Women should not be excluded from the process.

Dionisia: There are doctors who berate their patients. But it would be nice to actually have a dialogue.

Carmen: It's a slow process, but it's changing. Health practitioners need to change their mentality. But let's get back on topic. Who can remind me about the four pillars of the government's health policy?

Many Bartolinas were strong supporters of the Morales administration's "process of change" more broadly, but in this instance, the Ministry of Health event raised concerns for them about ongoing medical violence and the limits of reform. Victoria and Dionisia's refusal to avail themselves of health services clashed with Carmen's narrative about how Morales-era health reforms had enabled more culturally sensitive and participatory forms of care. The ministry official made some small concessions—yes, some doctors did their jobs badly—but she continually returned to how state health policies ultimately addressed the women's concerns. They should no longer fear giving birth in the health center, because now there were intercultural health policies and culturally adapted birthing rooms. They should no longer distance themselves from the health center, because now there was community participation.

For Sara Ahmed, "To be heard as complaining is to not be heard. To hear someone as complaining is an effective way of dismissing someone. You do not have to listen to the content of what she is saying if she is just complaining or always complaining" (2021, 1). Her words highlight how marking someone as a complainer—a category that is often racialized and gendered—can be a way to avoid engaging with what they have to say. In the Bolivian context, state officials somewhat expected community representatives to make complaints, understanding this practice to be in keeping with social movement engagement and the MAS's historical rise to power. At the same time, in participatory planning meetings, dismissing someone as a complainer became a way to retain the coherence of the narrative that state policies were still improving access to care and tuning in to the needs of Indigenous patients. Carmen could avoid engaging with Victoria's and Dionisia's critiques and continually attempt to bring the conversation back to the state's reforms and what they were trying to achieve.

Yet for participants themselves, complaint was a key mechanism for engaging the state. Most often, complaint was a means to draw attention to a problem—for example, the ongoing violence and extraction of biomedicine—and making demands for renewed material investment. Naomi Hossain (2010) emphasizes that what she calls "rude accountability" can be a strategy for marginalized citizens to demand public services, particularly in contexts in which formal mechanisms of accountability are few. Practices that may be perceived by others as "rude," including vocal expressions of complaint, criticism, and shaming, can exert social pressure on institutional actors to serve people better. I understand complaint to become a form of demanding accountability, especially amid the ruins of participatory development—when promises of "having a voice" had been extended since the 1990s, but when participation itself was often circumscribed and did not always lead to hoped-for changes. Several people I interviewed worried that their efforts to engage in formal participatory planning mechanisms had few results. Luisa, a former health committee member from a small village, described to me her frustrations. "We went to the municipal government with our project, with the list of our concerns, but they didn't do anything," she told me.

Given Carmen's deflections, it was also unclear whether public complaints would lead to being heard any more than going through official routes of proposal-making as Luisa had. But they became a key expression of frustration and pushing for more. Many community members hoped that representatives' complaints might nonetheless, to some extent, hold institutions accountable to their promises of transformed care.

WHEN DOCTORS MAKE COMPLAINTS

During the meeting in the village of R, after the NGO staffers had spoken, Dr. Wilmer gave a PowerPoint presentation to the gathered audience. His presentation focused primarily on vaccination coverage and health expenditures in the municipality over the past few months. When the presentation was over, Marcelino, a local representative from the CSUTCB, stood up. "Doctor," he said, his voice booming so that the entire room could hear. "We would like to know how many ambulances the hospital has."

"Two," Dr. Wilmer replied.

"Often, when we call, they tell us there's no ambulance available," Marcelino continued. "Several times when a woman was giving birth we wanted the ambulance to come—but, nothing."

Dr. Wilmer nodded, a little nervously. "The problem is that we have many accidents coming into the emergency room, because of the highway that runs through town. So often, our ambulances are rushing patients over to better-equipped hospitals in La Paz. Ideally, we would like to have more ambulances, including in the communities. It's in the works—more ambulances, more drivers, more contracts."

Participatory planning spaces were designed with the idea that community representatives could also hold local medical staff accountable. In this instance, a complaint about the condition of the ambulances also became a way to urge the hospital director to ensure that resources become available. What stood out to me about the encounter was that Dr. Wilmer, while somewhat nervously responding to the representative's question, also agreed that it would be valuable for the hospital to have more ambulances available. Over the course of many meetings, I observed how biomedical practitioners turned to grassroots representatives for support for their own litany of complaints and their own demands on the state. While biomedical practitioners occupied a position of authority, they also saw grassroots organizations as having a greater capacity to be heard, at both the municipal and state levels.

GHA staffers also directly sought to facilitate these forms of collaborative action. At a meeting to explain the elements of the SAFCI policy in the village of C, Mariela explained to the gathered group of community representatives and health center staff members the function of the Local Health Committee (*Comité Local de Salud*, CLS). The committee would be composed of representatives from the locally relevant grassroots organizations; they could both mobilize local community members to propose decisions and "hold the health personnel accountable if they fail to execute these plans." As she continued to describe the function of the CLS, Mariela also explained to the health care workers present that they could also rely on the CLS to help them make claims. She held up Ministry of Health–issued forms that health care workers were supposed to fill out with a list of expenses and a timeline for equipment that would need replacing. Turning to the health care providers, she clarified,

> These forms help us let the CLS know what's going on. They provide an explanation to the people. For example, for each injection we give we earn maybe two or three bolivianos. In other words, we don't get a lot of money from this. But we need money for things like gas. We usually end up paying this out of our pockets. The mayor needs to know about things like this. Sometimes, people think that we have a lot of money. But that's not how it is. The health center generates very little money. Maybe next year we'll be able to provide an official account for how our money is spent.

Later, after the group reconvened after lunch, the health personnel filled out the forms, guided by Mariela. Collectively, they filled out one form for keeping track of health care center equipment and how soon it would need to be replaced. She used the example of a desk to explain the timeline for its replacement: "Metal usually deteriorates in ten years, and wood in five."

A doctor in the audience spoke up, "We're missing a column detailing where the money comes from. Sometimes it comes from the municipality, an NGO, or us [out of our pockets]." He grinned and added jokingly, "We should send feedback to the ministry to let them know." The other health care workers in the audience laughed.

The joke was a moment of shared acknowledgment that requests for new equipment might also never be fulfilled. All the same, many biomedical providers strove to call community representatives' attention to ongoing problems in their health establishments. In Chapter 2, I described how a racialized politics of blame circulated in the hospital—in which providers' frequent focus on patients' ostensible unruliness and noncompliance obfuscated the material constraints shaping their work. But planning meetings also showed how points of alignment and shared political projects could emerge among providers and patients. These alignments especially came together around demanding material and infrastructural investments from the state that might facilitate care.

I observed Mariela's instructions on how to use forms and data being put into practice during a different municipal health meeting, this time held in the Machacamarca town hall. Dr. Wilmer stood before an audience of local union representatives. Pointing to budget numbers marked in red on his PowerPoint, he pleaded, "This is the amount of money the municipal government owes us. We don't have money for medications. Not even for thread for surgery. Our hands are tied, but you can help us."

Members of the audience murmured in consternation. When the doctor finished his presentation, several of them stood up to voice their support. The municipal representative for the Túpac Kataris announced that health should always come first and that his organization would draft a resolution in support of the hospital. Others countered, however, that they should wait until after the new mayor was sworn in to present him with their demands. The current mayor, they argued, had never done anything for the hospital.

For the staff of the cash-strapped Machacamarca Hospital, new "spaces of deliberation" became a key means of obtaining resources. As Dr. Wilmer's presentation indicated, the municipal government often failed to supply funds to the hospital—although it was required by law to spend 15.5 percent of its share of the national tax revenue on health care.[3] The hospital often lacked medications and supplies. Staffers were not paid for long stretches of time. Faced with precarious conditions, hospital personnel looked to alternative sources of support such as the Bartolina Sisas and Túpac Kataris, who they hoped could influence the municipal government. Despite limits to community participation, despite the fact that people's complaints were not always heard, biomedical providers understood social movement actors to still be politically powerful, to potentially have the ear of the MAS more than providers did. Complaint, then, could become a tenuous ground for building alliances—one that did not resolve all inequalities in the clinic but that nonetheless worked toward shared goals of appealing to institutions that might provide more funding and support.

ON THE POSSIBILITIES OF COMPLAINT

While officials sometimes met complaint with skepticism, I argue it constituted a central site of pushing for more from the state and generating possibilities for care beyond warm inclusion. As other scholars have noted, complaint, resentment, and contention can also be important strategies for engaging dominant institutions (Ahmed 2021; Coulthard 2014; Simpson 2014). Audra Simpson suggests that "thoughtful antagonism and 'contention' not 'reconciliation'" (2016, 3) becomes a key site for pushing back on settler colonial structures in the classroom and elsewhere; it operates not so much as an alternative to refusal (Simpson 2014) as a mode that exists alongside and in addition to it. In a similar vein, Glenn Coulthard understands Indigenous expressions of resentment and anger to "help prompt the very forms of self-affirmative praxis that generate rehabilitated Indigenous subjectivities and decolonized forms of life in ways that the combined politics of recognition and reconciliation has so far proven itself incapable of doing" (2014, 109).

Machacamarqueños' complaints both aligned with and diverged from other activist conversations about the radical restructuring of state institutions in Bolivia. Throughout this book, I have highlighted the challenges of enacting transformation through the colonial liberal state form—as decolonial projects were ultimately subsumed into a more general stance of warm care and inclusion. Thus, for a number of Indigenous activists and intellectuals in Bolivia, the state was a limited site of transformation. For Silvia Rivera Cusicanqui (2014), a key shortcoming of the Morales administration was its failure to reckon with how it was still part of an enduring colonial state apparatus. Others have also argued that a reversal of colonial orders is still inevitable, will still happen in the future, but that the MAS fell far short of this goal—a claim, for example, embraced by members of the Indianista student group, the Centro de Estudiantes Campesinos, that Marc Goodale (2019) interviewed. These discussions about the limitations of the MAS's decolonial project and the need for more radical reversals in the future also resonated with discussions about institutional transformation elsewhere. Their arguments also align with those in other contexts that highlight the inherent impossibility of decolonizing the settler state (TallBear 2019; Tuck and Yang 2012) and the ultimate need for "messy break up with the state—a rending not a reparation" (Shange 2019, 4). In Bolivia, calls for radical transformation emerged especially in a context in which colonial systems were continually reinventing themselves under the banner of decolonization.

In contrast, while complaints also centered on a call for the MAS to go further than it had, they also did not entail a complete disengagement from the state. Complaint, specifically, was a mode of continued engagement to strive to hold the state accountable—to strive to be heard, even if it meant sometimes being dismissed. Even so, I suggest, continued engagement through complaint was not entirely separate from activist calls for abolishing or radically restructuring the state. Indigenous and campesino communities in Bolivia engaged in multiple, sometimes overlapping modes of reckoning with the colonial state and working to push institutions further. Complaints were also continuous with other forms of political action, including protests in the form of marches, strikes, and road blockades; they often laid the groundwork for further action.

With this in mind, I understand complaint to be a lively practice of critique. Reflections on academic practices of critique have highlighted the value of analyzing relations of power, as well as the potential pitfalls of focusing narrowly on critique. Critiques of colonial state systems can sometimes treat them as overly fixed and totalizing (Lambert 2022)—and simply articulating critiques of power does not always lead to transforming those relations of power. Notably, as Sara Ahmed points out, institutional actors can also deploy statements that are antiracist and critique the workings of power; yet many of these speech acts are fundamentally "nonperformative"—that is, "they do not do what they say: they do not, as it were, commit a person, organization, or state to an action" (2006, 104). Yet when mobilized as part of a lived, everyday praxis, articulating public critiques became a way to both render visible policy shortcomings and refigure social relations in ways that sought to commit institutions to action.

Practices of complaint, moreover, ultimately raised questions about care as a site of state-led political transformation. In some respects, complaints made by my interlocutors during community health meetings were also demands for better care—to urge the state to invest in health services and sustain well-being. But they also complicated the promise of care—or at least, rejected the notion that warm affects and promises of inclusion would necessarily translate to better care.

Scholars have likewise called for attention to care's "non-innocent genealogies" (Murphy 2015) and highlighted how the "ruse of repair" (Stuelke 2021) can also replicate neoliberal models of change. Such critiques are not a blanket rejection of care, which, as others have emphasized, can also sometimes be an important site of political resistance and potentiality.[4] But as tracing Bolivian state health policies shows, some iterations of institutional care can also foreclose or deflect change. We might think back to the encounter with Carmen, when she invoked promises of warm care as a way to not hear Victoria and Dionisia's complaints. Or we might think back even further, to Chapter 1, when Alonzo likewise sought to deflect healers' complaints and emphasize all that the state was doing to build inclusion and participation. Complaint was a way of rejecting the state's emphasis on warm care, of saying, "This is not enough."

Complaint was not always effective; it did not always directly lead to the results that people hoped for. Complaint was a "rude" practice (Hossain 2010) that took shape amid the ruins of decades of participatory development, when promises of having a voice in policy were often circumscribed or did not lead to material changes. Still, practices of complaining both within and outside of spaces designated for participation were a central step toward holding the state accountable to its promises of good living. As I have shown throughout this book, patients, healers, and other residents of Machacamarca understood the state to be responsible to the body through health care—a responsibility that might variably be understood in terms of redistribution, personalized attention and obligation, and long-term care. Complaint became a ground for reshuffling relations, especially when these obligations did not come through. Sometimes, it could generate tenuous alliances and forms of solidarity between providers and patients; when a racialized politics of blame often pitted providers against patients, complaint could be leveraged to highlight the linked struggles of both groups. Other times, it became a means of reminding state, nonprofit, and medical institutions that they needed to be accountable to the people that they served, particularly given the MAS's own roots in a productive politics of contention, complaint, and protest. Complaint rendered visible limitations of promises of participation and warm care and demanded that institutions do more.

———

I began this book with the story of Violeta who, as she sat in the hospital waiting room, joked about doctors not speaking Aymara while sitting under a sign that welcomed patients to the hospital in Aymara. In a small way, her humorous remarks might also be understood as a form of complaint—as a way of calling attention to what was promised but had not yet come to fruition. Complaint threaded through many of the encounters I describe in this book, as my interlocutors expressed frustrations with the limitations of care.

State officials, as I described in Chapter 1, crafted narratives and expectations of change around their decolonial projects—expectations that later also became central to many Machacamarqueños' complaints. Some changes to the health care system did take shape—yet were often not enough to counter deeply entrenched, colonial and racialized systems of intervention. Yet while complaint was an important part of the history of social movements and of the MAS, many state officials also came to see practices of complaint as unruly and unproductive. They also expressed skepticism in the face of complaint—or, along with NGO workers, sought to channel demands into what they deemed more feasible ways of talking about health.

Still, for many patients and residents of Machacamarca, complaint opened up different forms of obligation, care, and accountability. Very often, they made complaints and demands in terms of material and infrastructural investment. At the same time, these were not simply demands for more development; infrastructure was also bound up in other hopes for long-term attention and dignified living. In a context in which health care continued to fall short, complaint through community participation became a way to demand more from the state.

CONCLUSION
POLITICAL AFTERMATHS

IN MARCH 2020, COVID-19 CAME to Bolivia. Machacamarca was a small early hotspot of the pandemic, and the hospital was quickly overwhelmed. State officials made several highly publicized arrests of townsfolk who had thrown a large party, although the party had occurred before the official lockdown banning such gatherings. Photographs appeared in the press of police in hazmat suits carrying away the *pasantes* (sponsors of the party) and the mayor to prison. As state officials formally enacted a national lockdown, new images began to circulate in the press: those of police going after farmers breaking lockdown to harvest potatoes in the rural Altiplano.

As I talked on the phone with my compadre as we each went into our respective lockdowns—I in Southern California, he in Machacamarca—he worried about not having enough to eat, about not earning enough money from selling at the market. He wondered, is this sickness happening because of Jeanine Añez? If Evo hadn't been ousted, this wouldn't have happened.

DOUBLE CRISIS, DOUBLE PANDEMIC

On November 12, 2019, some months before the Covid-19 pandemic hit, Evo Morales resigned from the presidency. He had recently declared victory in the October 19 national elections, which would grant him a fourth term in office. Yet a pause in the vote counting (as the system switched over from the preliminary vote-counting mechanism to the official vote-counting mechanism) prompted opposition groups to accuse him of fraud. Growing protests against his alleged fraud ballooned into a police mutiny and, eventually, a televised demand from the leader of the armed forces that the president resign. Faced with mounting pressure, Evo Morales, his vice president, and other top administration officials resigned and eventually sought refuge in Mexico. Then, in a nearly empty legislative chamber—absent members of the majority MAS party—opposition legislators selected conservative politician Jeanine Añez to become interim president of Bolivia (Claros 2022; Farthing and Becker 2021; Valdivia Rivera 2021).

During her year-long presidency, Añez and members of her administration pursued a punitive agenda. In November 2019, shortly after she assumed office, she authorized the use of military force. After she signed the authorization decree, armed forces massacred a total of twenty-two protestors at Senkata (in El Alto) and Sacaba (near Cochabamba). Añez appointed Arturo Murillo as her interior minister, who quickly set up a task force with the goal of pursuing "seditious" actors and former MAS officials (Claros 2022; Farthing and Becker 2021; Valdivia Rivera 2021). Many of my interlocutors described Añez's presidency as a time of intensified repression, conflict, fear, and racism. One of my neighbors in Machacamarca, for example, described how she had ultimately decided to leave her job working as an *empleada* (maid) in La Paz. She recounted that in the early days after Morales's ouster, she and other Aymara women were called racist names and had objects thrown at them when going to work in the Zona Sur (the upper-class district of La Paz).

It was in this climate of increased repression and conflict that the Covid pandemic arrived in Bolivia. In March 2020, President Añez's administration enacted a strict lockdown to contain the virus. Bolivians were allowed to leave their homes only on certain days of the week for groceries and supplies, based on the last digit of their government-issued ID card. Only one member of each household was allowed to leave each day. Members of the military patrolled the streets and fined those who left their homes on days they were not permitted to do so (Alderman 2020; Velasco Guachalla et al. 2021.). The Añez administration's emergency decree instating a strict lockdown often became the grounds for further pursuing punitive action. Military and police were positioned as the protagonists of the "war" against Covid-19, who were to imprison those who broke quarantine or did not wear a mask (Gustafson 2021). Strict measures were couched in fear-mongering discourse—simultaneously emphasizing the terrifying nature of the virus and placing blame for its transmission on irresponsible individuals (Pachaguaya Yujra and Terrazas Sosa 2020). Yet if Bolivian officials initially put in place strict measures, they also did little to support people through the lockdown. In a country where the informal sector made up a large portion of economic activity, and where there continued to be high levels of poverty, the lockdown measures were devastating for many. As my compadre and others put it, they feared they would not be able to feed their families. State economic relief might have helped mitigate these effects—but the onetime payment of 500 bolivianos (about 71.50 USD) per family did little to alleviate pressures (Farthing and Becker 2021).

Although a lockdown—combined with sufficient economic support and social protection—can be an important measure for slowing the spread of a pandemic, in Bolivia the state's Covid mitigation policies had limited success. The Bolivian NGO Boligráfica, which published data throughout the pandemic, pointed out that Covid deaths were likely undercounted (Foronda and UDAPE 2023). Factoring in excess deaths (from statistical analysis of the average yearly death rate) put Bolivia's pandemic death toll in 2020 as one of the highest in the world (Trigo, Kurmanaev, and McCann 2020). My social media feeds overflowed with pleas for help finding hospital beds and ventilators at multiple points in 2020 and early 2021. The country's health care system, as I have detailed throughout this book, had long faced many challenges of resource and infrastructural shortages and warranted distrust of biomedical care provision—that would have made tackling a pandemic a difficult task for whomever held the presidency. But the Añez administration's combination of punitive approaches and general mismanagement exacerbated what was already going to be a challenging situation. Her minister of health, Marcelo Navajas, also became embroiled in a scandal after whistleblowers leaked that he had been pocketing money from the purchase of faulty ventilators (Velasco Guachalla et al. 2021). Covid-19 compounded what was already a devastating political crisis in Bolivia—what many ended up calling a "double pandemic" or a "double crisis"—as political violence and violence of the pandemic converged.

These events highlight how many of the dynamics I have described in this book—including resource constraints, the racialization of care, the pathologization of Indigenous subjects, and the intertwining of benevolence and violence—were intensified during the Covid-19 pandemic. During Añez's administration, medical violence intersected with state violence in new ways, as the police enforced quarantine and arrested ostensible rule breakers, and as the death toll kept rising because of material shortages. While there are continuities in colonial projects across administrations, the interim government rearticulated them and leveraged them in increasingly devastating ways.

After multiple delays, the Añez administration—intended to be an interim caretaker government—called for new elections to occur in October 2020. The MAS put forward Luis Arce, the former minister of the economy under Morales, as candidate for president, and David Choquehuanca, an Aymara movement activist and former minister of foreign relations under Morales, as their slate. The October elections went smoothly, and Arce won by a landslide, presenting at the time a renewed sense of hope for many of my interlocutors (Díaz Cuellar 2022).

Arce sought to return to the more progressive social policies that characterized the MAS. Yet his administration has also faced numerous challenges, including increased divisions and political battles

within the MAS, a less favorable global economic climate, and an ongoing Covid-19 pandemic. The Arce administration stated that it would
prioritize reinvesting in universal health care and pandemic management (Booth 2020). Hesitant to enact another lockdown, the Ministry of
Health instead emphasized masking and vaccination as key strategies
in 2021 and 2022, slowly cobbling together vaccines from the WHO,
Russia, and China. Arce's administration formally ended the national
sanitary emergency in July 2023 (EFE 2023). Still, health care policies
continued to encounter challenges like resource inequalities (especially when it came to access to vaccines) and uneven infrastructures.

WARM CARE AND REINSCRIPTION

This book has centrally examined the question of how and why, during
Evo Morales's presidency, state officials' projects to decolonize health
care ended up reinscribing colonial conditions of care. I have shown
how channeling proposals for change through existing liberal and colonial biopolitical forms limited their capacity to constitute a radical
break. Specifically, warm care emerged as a predominating framework as policymakers shifted away from decolonial proposals for ontological pluralism, dignified living, and material redistribution and
instead embraced an emphasis on kind, humane, inclusive, and equal
treatment for Indigenous patients.

Warm care could sometimes open up new avenues for Indigenous
patients, who leveraged it for different ends when pursuing biomedical courses of treatment. A patient's husband could demand his rights
to be present during the birth of his child. A partera might teach an
intern how to give a patient massages. Patients might observe who was
an attentive doctor and rope them into deeper relations of obligation.
But very often, it also extended continuities with colonial projects and
modes of intervention. Biomedical practitioners, for example, came
to tie warmth to treating all patients equally—but did so in ways that
replicated racial hierarchies in the clinic (Chapter 2). NGO projects
to build warm birthing rooms did not displace authoritative biomedical interventions or obstetric violence (Chapter 3). Warm care also

became linked, differently, to projects to bureaucratize community-based care—under which state promises of visibility and inclusion, shored up through playful mapping projects, also erased interpersonal obligations among providers and patients (Chapter 5). Warm care, across many sites, became a way to urge commensuration and collaboration with dominant biomedical norms.

These reinscriptions did not occur in a vacuum. As I show throughout this book, they were also conditioned by historically rooted unequal national and global resource flows. Bolivian state projects to resolve the problem of funding, in turn, depended on ongoing resource capitalism and extraction—and did not always bring about the material investments in health care that some hoped for. When it came to health care, enduring liberal and biopolitical modes of intervention remained entangled in questions of what projects got funded, what policy enactments were possible amid resource constraints, and who ended up doing the work of care. As I described in Chapters 3 and 4, warm care also depended on the racialized and gendered labor of Indigenous traditional healers and midwives, brought into clinics under paradigms of inclusion. Simultaneously, warm care deflected attention from the ongoing racial, gendered, and material inequalities at work in medical settings.

Yet if modes of institutionalized warm care—centered on making difference manageable and commensurate—often foreclosed political transformation, Machacamarqueños also rerouted care into novel forms. For many patients and healers, care was also a matter of fulfilling social obligations and crafting accountability across hierarchies. They sought to bring biomedical practitioners working at the local hospital into kin relations—and also ultimately sought to bring the state into relations of ethical redistribution and obligation. Such practices, unfolding within local moral worlds and norms of care, both engaged and subverted state projects of reform. Healers, for example, participated actively in the bureaucratic and labor regimes they hoped would grant them visibility and legitimacy in the eyes of the state, but they also rearticulated state promises of redistribution as a state obligation to care for the very relations that might sustain healing and well-being.

In turn, when patients sought to make biomedical providers kin, they sought to craft new forms of biomedical practice that might be more efficacious through its attention to relations. These practices often maintained social hierarchies and could also create new burdens for providers as well as patients. But as Machacamarqueños were at turns critical and hopeful about the capacity of state and medical institutions to deliver what they understood to be good care, they sought to reroute institutional projects into more livable forms.

When state promises of transformation did not come through, many residents of Machacamarca turned to making complaints, especially in spaces designated for community-based participatory planning and deliberation. Understanding complaint to be a generative practice of critique, I have highlighted how it became a method for exposing the limits of reform and demanding accountability from institutions. If complaints were sometimes dismissed, they nonetheless became small steps toward transforming relationships among patients, providers, and governmental institutions. Centering dissatisfaction, contention, and disruption, practices of complaint rejected the tenets of warm care that promised sympathy and inclusion. Instead, they laid the groundwork for building health care that might be more responsive and more accountable to social movement demands.

DECOLONIZING MEDICINE, PUBLIC HEALTH, AND GLOBAL HEALTH

These conversations about the possibilities and limits of institutional decolonization have ever more relevance, especially given the growing interest among global health scholars in engaging questions of decolonization. Beginning in 2020, a spate of publications started emerging in English-language medical journals calling for the decolonization of global health.[1] These discussions emerged in part in response to the profound inequalities of the Covid-19 pandemic (and the Ebola epidemic before it), as well as growing protests for racial justice and against police violence in the United States in the wake of George Floyd's murder (Herrick and Bell 2022; Krugman 2023). Scholars writing in academic journal articles embraced a range of proposals for addressing the historical and ongoing structures of inequality that have shaped global health as a field. Some emphasized the importance of epistemic decolonization and challenging the centrality of Eurocentric modes of knowledge (Affun-Adegbulu and Adegbulu 2020). Others turned their focus to material resource flows and unequal relationships between Global North and Global South, particularly as centers in the Global North continue to be main sites of global health funding and dominant knowledge production (Lawrence and Hirsch 2020).

Still, critiques have also started to emerge within these conversations—particularly as more global health and development agencies have deployed the term "decolonization." Daniel Krugman (2023), for example, argues that proposals for decolonization in global health have increasingly been subject to what Olúfẹ́mi O. Táíwò (2022) calls "elite capture" in which powerful institutions might appropriate the concept to maintain their own interests, but also largely evacuate it of its radical meanings. Uses of the term "decolonization" in the global health policy world often echo the trends that Eve Tuck and Wayne Yang (2012) described over a decade ago in their influential article, "Decolonization Is Not a Metaphor." They worried people were increasingly taking the term "decolonization" to be generically equivalent to any project of social justice instead of entailing the return of stolen lands to Indigenous nations. Building on this earlier work, recent critiques have pointed out that while tackling the historically rooted and structural inequalities of global health is an important goal, institutional appropriations of the term "decolonization" have often sidestepped that very goal.

Notably, neither proposals for decolonizing global health nor critiques of their limitations have cited or engaged with the Bolivian state's over-a-decade-long experiment in decolonizing medicine and public health. Bolivian health policy reforms point to the challenges and complexities of enacting substantive transformation within dominant institutions. For some of my interlocutors, as well as some activists and scholars in Bolivia, there is no enacting decolonial change through the colonial state (Rivera Cusicanqui 2014). Transformation, to echo Fausto Reinaga (1969), would entail a "struggle of national liberation" (442, my translation) and remaking institutions from the ground up. My findings lead me to agree with perspectives that state (and NGO and global agency) capture offers a limited site of transformation, given the ways that these institutions have been and continue to be built around colonial projects. Simultaneously, I acknowledge and center the ways that many of my interlocutors have engaged in actions to make institutional encounters work for them, or sought to hold institutional actors accountable, including in ways that aligned with anticolonial goals. The latter perspectives are not entirely incompatible with the former but highlight how the work of transformation might take shape in multiple ways, across multiple sites.

While there are no clear or easy fixes, dwelling on the limits of policy reform highlights the importance of engaging with the work that policy recipients are already doing to create habitable worlds, including in ways that challenge or complicate dominant modes of fixing and governing life. As I described across multiple chapters, state, NGO, and medical actors often positioned illness as originating within Indigenous bodies, households, and cultural practices—understanding these to be continued sites of regulation and improvement. They also often flattened the dynamism and complexity of practices around health, healing, and care and instead expected adherence to a predetermined narrative of fixed cultural difference. But, as residents of Machacamarca worked to pull medical and state workers into relations of ethical obligation, they also troubled neat distinctions at the core of colonial biopolitics and foregrounded how care providers and recipients were already imbricated in each other's lives. Through practices like kin-making and complaint, they sought to create more accountable—and livable—forms of care.

Simultaneously, complaint also emerged out of a refusal to be satisfied with current conditions. Conversations with my interlocutors—as well as other activists and writers in Bolivia—were a continual reminder that anticolonial action required a deeper project of structural undoing. Structures rooted in both national and global colonialism and capitalism—including racism and racialization, gender inequality, labor exploitation, and land dispossession—were still at the heart of inequalities in the health care system, shaping both the incidence of illness and how institutions engaged in care. If policymakers frequently named colonialism and capitalism as concerns, warm care, as both a discourse and a practice, often served to obfuscate the workings of structural inequalities and maintain the functioning of the existing health care system. The Morales administration's health policies were a small step toward transforming conditions of care—but they were also not the final say. Still, as many in Bolivia have noted, that the current system will always exist is not a foregone conclusion.[2] Possibilities for undoing, remaking, and, ultimately, decolonization, are always still on the horizon.

ACKNOWLEDGMENTS

This book was first and foremost made possible by the many people in Bolivia who took the time to talk to me and share meals with me and who allowed me to accompany them as they both sought and provided care. As I write about care, I am continually reminded that the care that people showed me was central to bringing this book into the world. Because of the sensitive nature of health and illness experiences—as well as ongoing struggles over resources and compensation in the hospital—I have anonymized the names of most of my interlocutors, as well as the name of the town, hospital, and NGO that figure centrally into the book. But while I cannot name individuals, I hope I can at least begin to acknowledge the many debts I owe to those who took part in this project.

I owe an enormous debt to the many patients, town residents, and community leaders in Bolivia who shared with me their experiences of health, illness, and navigating the health care system. Sharing such experiences can be a vulnerable act, opening up feelings of frustration, pain, and humor, as well as hope. I am humbled by people's willingness to share their stories with me. I am also deeply grateful to both the biomedical and traditional medical providers who talked to me about the challenges of their work. Their narratives of labor precarity and efforts to provide care under constrained circumstances helped me to understand the multiple layers involved in building a more just health care system. Finally, this book also would not have been possible without the many Bolivian state bureaucrats and NGO workers who shared with me their desires, hopes, and work in transforming the health care system, even as they encountered many limitations and challenges. I owe a particular thank you to the nonprofit organization that I anonymize as "Global Health Aid," or "GHA," in the manuscript, which put me in touch with hospital administrators, state officials, and many others who would become essential to this project.

I continue to learn from many of my interlocutors who have encouraged me to think through both the possibilities and limits of state-led change, as well as the potential of complaint and critique in holding institutions accountable. I hope I have done justice to the complexity of struggles around health care in Bolivia—and any mistakes or omissions in this book are my own.

I began work on this project at Yale University, where I encountered a vibrant intellectual community that continually challenged me to become a better scholar. Marcia Inhorn took on the role of my committee chair when I returned to New Haven after completing my ethnographic research in Bolivia; I am grateful for her guidance and her pushing me to think about the broader implications of my work. Sean Brotherton, who was my advisor for many years before he left Yale, continued to support my project as an external committee member. His insights on questions of politics, the state, and the body continue to stay with me. Kalyanakrishnan Sivaramakrishnan shaped my thinking about questions of the state and development projects; his continual feedback and careful reading of my work showed him to be an exceptional mentor. Joanna Radin, lending a historian's perspective, helped me to think more robustly about the relationships between colonialism, public and global health, and everyday medical practice. I am also grateful to have learned from and received feedback on early versions of the project from Jafari Allen, Kamari Clarke, Karen Nakamura, and Sarah Schneiderman.

At Yale, I am especially thankful for my graduate school cohort—

Samar Al-Bulushi, Nilay Erten, Sahana Ghosh, Ryan Jobson, Caroline Merrifield, and Sayd Randle—as we exchanged drafts, shared ideas, and provided insights on each other's work. My work also benefitted from the insights of others, including Sarah Brothers, Andra Chastain, Gavriel Cutipa-Zorn, Alder Keleman Saxena, Tess Lanzarotta, Catherine Mas, Jess Newman, Haesoo Park, Marco Ramos, and Naomi Sussman. Long after we graduated, Sayd Randle continued to read multiple chapters of this book. Her incisive feedback—as well as her continual friendship and support—helped bring this manuscript into being.

I wrote and revised much of this book as a new faculty member at Scripps College. I am extraordinarily lucky to be a member of what our students have called a "small but mighty" three-person Anthropology department. My colleagues, Lara Deeb and Seo Young Park, are inspirational scholars and mentors. From day one, they provided me with guidance on research, teaching, and navigating the challenges of the job. Both also read a full draft of the book manuscript, providing invaluable commentary that shaped this work.

At Scripps, I have also been fortunate to encounter colleagues across the disciplines who have helped create a community of support and solidarity. My thanks especially to Claudia Arteaga, Leila Mansouri, and Martín Vega, who have directly and indirectly shaped this project in various forms.

As part of the Claremont Colleges Consortium, I am also privileged to be part of a wider vibrant intercollegiate Anthropology program that has included Cristina Bejarano, Ángela Castillo Ardila, Emily Chao, Marianne De Laet, Cécile Evers, Joanne Nucho, Daniel Segal, Omer Shah, and Claudia Strauss. As I was finishing the book, I formed a writing group with Cristina, Ángela, and Cécile, who offered helpful suggestions on sections of the manuscript.

This manuscript also benefitted from in-depth comments from Felicity Aulino and Pamela Calla, who dedicated a full day to leading a workshop on the full draft of the manuscript. Their brilliant and insightful feedback helped shape the book into what it is today. At various stages, this book also benefitted from commentary on chapters and related articles from numerous others, including Martha Lincoln,

Nicole Rosner, Sonia Rupcic, Lana Salman, Seda Saluk, Aalyia Sarrudin, and Emily Yates-Doerr.

Dylan Kyung-lim White at Stanford University Press has been a fantastic editor. His early enthusiasm for the project, his insights on style and framing, and his continual support throughout the process have been invaluable. At Stanford UP, Austin Michael Araujo also helped with the logistics of the manuscript and answered many of my questions. Gigi Mark and members of the production team shepherded this project to completion. I am also incredibly grateful to the two anonymous reviewers of this manuscript, whose crucial commentary helped this book take its final form.

The research and writing of this book was supported by numerous grants, including the National Science Foundation's Doctoral Dissertation Improvement Grant, the American Council of Learned Society's Graves Award in the Humanities, the Reed Foundation's Ruth Landes Memorial Research Fund, the Tinker Foundation's Field Research Grant, numerous summer research grants from Yale University and Scripps College, and a sabbatical research award from Scripps College. I also received writing support as a selected participant in the Ann Johnson Institute's 2023 Writing Retreat with the theme of "Medicine, Technology, and Marginalized Populations." The retreat not only gave me time and motivation to write, but also introduced me to an incredible community of interdisciplinary scholars.

Portions of Chapter 3, "Warm and Cold: Cultural Adaptation and the Circulation of Temperature," were previously published in *Medical Anthropology Quarterly* as an article titled "There Is No Place Like Home: Imitation and the Politics of Recognition in Bolivian Obstetric Care."

In Bolivia, the staff at the National Archives and Library in Sucre and at the Historical Archives of La Paz helped me locate key historical documents, including policy texts and medical review articles. Jaime Mejía, my Aymara instructor in La Paz, was a wonderful teacher. I am also grateful for coffees, meals, and conversations over the years with other scholars working in Bolivia, including Ana María Aguilar, Alissa Bernstein, Kate Centellas, Susan Ellison, Nicole Fabricant, Bret

Gustafson, Brian Johnson, Pedro Portugal, Nancy Postero, and Maria Tapias. These conversations have profoundly shaped my thinking on questions of politics, health care, and indigeneity in Bolivia.

I also am thankful for the research assistants who helped with various components of this project. In La Paz, Varinia Asuncion and Justina Luna transcribed my interviews. At Scripps, my student assistant, Jennifer Rufino, helped to organize bibliographic sources and archival documents.

Long before I began writing this book, my professors at the University of Arizona set me on the path to becoming an anthropologist. Brian Silverstein's Cultural Anthropology course in Spring 2007 inspired my interest in the field, and he continued to mentor me in later courses and on my undergraduate thesis project. Mark Nichter's seminar in Medical Anthropology first introduced me to graduate study in an area that would become my intellectual home, while Diane Austin's mentorship through the Bureau of Applied Research in Anthropology taught me many of the skills I would later use in ethnographic research. Without their early guidance, this book would not exist.

I am grateful for the care and support of my extended family in Bolivia, including my many cousins and especially my aunts and uncles who opened their homes to me many times over the years: Rolando and Michele, Beatriz and Pablo, Juan Antonio and Cécile, Luly and Pepe. Beatriz, Pablo, and Pepe passed away before this book was published, and I hold them in my heart always.

Finally, I thank my parents, Jorge and Silvia, my brother, Nicolas, and my sister-in-law, Mariana, for their unwavering support. My family's kindness and consideration for others, their intellectual curiosity, and their interest in politics and in the world helped shape me into the person I am today. Throughout a long and often arduous writing process, they listened to me work through ideas and lent their emotional support as I hammered out chapter drafts. I could not have written this book without them.

NOTES

Introduction: Waiting for Reform

1. I use pseudonyms for the name of the town, the hospital, NGOs, and all individuals who are not known public figures. Anonymizing was a difficult decision, because many people I interviewed would have liked to see their town name in print. Moreover, towns and the land they are situated on have specific histories, and the use of pseudonyms can also have a deracinating effect. However, given the infrastructural and labor challenges faced by the local municipal hospital and the sometimes-sensitive nature of patient and practitioner experiences, I felt it important to follow anthropological convention in this case and de-identify people, place names, and institutions as much as possible. "Machacamarca" simply means "New Town" in Aymara, and it is the actual, commonly used place name of numerous towns and neighborhoods across the Altiplano. Long ago, the area where I conducted research was also called "Machacamarca" before the river changed course, houses were moved, and a new name was adopted. "New Town," although in some ways generic, gestures both to a situated history and to a current context of rapid rural urbanization.

2. The Aymara are one of the largest Indigenous groups in Bolivia, with approximately 1,191,352 members (Centro de Documentación e Información Bolivia 2013).

3. For example, Lucia Guerra-Reyes' (2019) account of intercultural birthing policies in Peru describes the common use of the phrase *calidad con calidez* (quality with warmth). In Bolivia, this phrase was also used, although I more commonly heard the formulation *con calidad y calidez* (with quality and

warmth). Although slightly different in their phrasing, both point to notions that medical rigor ("quality") should be combined with warmth, especially in contexts in which managing Indigenous cultural difference became a central concern.

4. On health policy and inequalities in Latin America, see Andaya 2014; Berry 2010; Briggs and Mantini-Briggs 2003, 2016; Guerra-Reyes 2019; Jarrín 2017; Vega 2018; Yates-Doerr 2015. For discussions of neoliberalism and health, see Abadía-Barrero 2022; Han 2012; Martínez 2018; Tapias 2015.

5. Charles Briggs and Clara Mantini-Briggs (2016, 171) similarly point out in conversation with their Warao interlocutors that narratives about the origins and temporality of disease reflect positioned ways of knowing. For at least some of the Warao, illness begins not with the onset of symptoms, but with the negative effects of colonialism following the arrival of Christopher Columbus.

6. While some scholars have argued that land dispossession, rather than labor exploitation, is the central mechanism of settler colonialism, others have troubled this distinction. I follow Shannon Speed (2017) and Bianet Castellanos (2017), who have argued that land dispossession and labor exploitation are complexly interrelated processes in the context of Latin American settler colonialism. Their arguments also echo those put forward by Aymara Katarista activists who, in the 1970s in Bolivia, centered the uneven co-constitution of ethnicity and class (see Dangl 2019; Sanjinés 2004).

7. While dynamics of colonialism and capitalism should not be conflated (Liboiron 2021), they have often gone hand-in-hand, historically shaping one another's trajectories (Ramones and Merry 2021).

8. For works on coloniality, see Castro-Gómez 2005; Espinosa Miñoso 2022; Lugones 2007; Maldonado-Torres 2007; Mendoza 2020; Mignolo 2012; Moraña, Dussel, and Jáuregui 2008; Quijano 1999; 2000; Segato 2013; 2016.

9. On *mestizaje* in Bolivia and the Andean region more broadly, see de la Cadena 2000; Molina 2021; Ravindran 2020; 2021; Rivera Cusicanqui 1984.

10. There has been some debate among scholars thinking with and about Indigenous critiques how to best describe the long-term, lingering, and reentrenching effects of European colonialism. Scholars working in the Americas have at times critiqued the use of the term "postcolonial," first developed by subaltern studies scholars, many situated in recently decolonized, former franchise colonies in the mid-twentieth century. Critics have argued that "postcolonial" implies an "after" that is not well applied in contexts of long-term European settlement where the colonizers never left (Klor de Alva 1992). At the same time, scholars who do engage with the term have articulated a nuanced take on the "post-" in "postcolonial," arguing that it is not so much about a clear before and after as the ways that domination has taken on new and different forms in context (cf. Hall 1996). In the context of enduring Anglo

colonialism (e.g., the United States, Canada, Australia, New Zealand) the term "settler colonialism" is often used to describe processes of European settlement on land and simultaneous project of elimination of Indigenous peoples (Coulthard 2014; Simpson 2014; Wolfe 2006). Some scholars also apply this term to Latin American contexts—which share broadly similar patterns of long-term settlement, and where one might also draw important lines of continuity beyond contemporary nation-state borders (Castellanos 2017; Saldaña-Portillo 2016; Speed 2017). Others, however, have cautioned against the way that growing use of this term displaces ways that scholars in Latin America and its diaspora have long written about "coloniality" (*colonialidad*) to describe colonial reinscriptions (see Lugones 2007; Mignolo 2012; Quijano 1999), as well as specific differences in ways that Iberian colonialism had operated in these contexts. Others, still, point out that writings from Latin America on coloniality—which have gained global scholarly traction—are primarily from white and mestizo men, and have often failed to cite earlier writings pointing to similar processes on "internal colonialism" (*colonialismo interno*) (González Casanovas 1965; Rivera Cusicanqui 2010). These concerns raise questions about the terms on which academic terminology circulates and gains traction (Pérez-Bustos 2017). In an effort to think with these different genealogies, as well as how technologies of domination travel across contexts, I use the broader term "colonialism" (*colonialismo*) in this book, while attending to the specificity of the ways it continues to be rearticulated through the Bolivian state.

11. Growing academic conversations on colonialism and decolonization in medicine have focused heavily on the aftermaths of European and U.S. administrative colonialisms and their relevance for global health, highlighting how historically rooted structures continue to shape conditions of knowledge production and medical resource flows between Global North and Global South. Yet as Anpotowin Jensen and Victor Lopez-Carmen (2022) have argued, these discussions of colonialism in global health often ignore the experiences of Indigenous nations and how health care systems intersect with enduring settlement-based colonialisms. In my analysis, I foreground both the dynamics of state-based colonialism and the coloniality of global health, understanding these dynamics to also intersect in complex ways.

12. Spanish colonists used the term *Indio* (Indian) to classify the original inhabitants of the land they colonized. The term *Indígena* (Indigenous) also started to be used in Bolivian legislation by the early nineteenth century. Over several centuries, the meaning of both categories—as defined within state and legal documents—shifted, variably linked to a person's geographic location, occupation, or language use (Arigho-Stiles 2024; Barragán 2011). After the 1952 national revolution, the Bolivian state sought to unite the nation around a

234 NOTES TO THE INTRODUCTION

shared mestizo identity and shed ethnic identifiers in favor of the class-based term *campesino* (peasant). Later, with anticolonial social movement activism beginning in the 1970s, the global rise of an Indigenous rights framework in the 1980s and 1990s, and the eventual recognition of Bolivia as a "multicultural nation" in the 1994 Bolivian constitution, the term *Indígena* came to the fore again, often in association with emancipatory struggles (Postero 2007).

13. The English-language term "care" offers an imperfect translation of multiple ways that my interlocutors talked about providing for others. In Aymara, the verb *uywaña* might be translated as "care," but more accurately means to rear, nurture, and grow in relation; it is taken up less in the context of the clinic and more in the context of mutual care between human and non-human others in a sentient rural landscape. In Spanish, two words are often used. The first, *cuidar*, is closest to the English "care" and is often used as imperative *te cuidas* (take care) or for the act of taking care of another (*cuidar a alguien*). Second is the term *atención*, which is more along the lines of "service" but is used to describe institutional health care (*la atención en salud*) and care for a patient (*atender a un paciente*). When patients described their local hospital as a place *donde no hay atención* (where there is no treatment/care), they frequently pointed to the intertwining of bureaucratic and material with affective demands. Given this variation of terms, I attend to both the specificity and multiplicity of ways that patients, providers, and bureaucrats weigh questions of who should be provided for and how.

14. On care as a moral, embodied practice, see also Buch 2018; Kleinman 2007; Mol 2008; Mol, Moser, and Pols 2015.

15. Anthropologists who have written about the *kharikhari* (or *karisiri* or *pishtaco*) have frequently emphasized the importance of fat to Aymara and Quechua ontologies of the body, personhood, and well-being. Fat is the main source of one's vitality and is constituted through social relations (Canessa 2012; Crandon-Malamud 1991). The fact that some of my interlocutors were suggesting that the kharikhari might steal blood instead was a recent conceptual shift (and not something upon which everyone agreed). My sense was that this shift emerged from increasing encounters with hospital biomedicine, as well as broader transformations in social norms and approaches to healing that accompanied rural urbanization in municipalities like Machacamarca.

16. Abimbola and Pai 2020; Affun-Adegbulu and Adegbulu 2020; Büyüm et al. 2020; Herrick and Bell 2022; Lawrence and Hirch 2020; Richardson 2020.

17. I am focusing primarily on highland Aymara and Quechua decolonial theory in this work because they share a context with many of my interlocutors and were also highly influential for how the MAS articulated its project. Nonetheless, this excludes a range of decolonial perspectives and work also coming from Indigenous communities in the Bolivian lowlands.

18. As a share of total government expenditure, health care spending increased over the course of the Morales administration from 8.75 percent in 2006 to 13.67 percent in 2019 according to Our World in Data (https://ourworldindata.org/grapher/health-expenditure-government-expenditure?tab=chart&country=BOL). As a percentage of GDP, health care spending increased from 4.66 percent in 2006 to 6.92 percent in 2019 (https://ourworldindata.org/grapher/total-healthcare-expenditure-gdp?tab=chart&country=BOL).

19. On care's radical potential, see Dokumaci 2020; Finch 2022; Grande 2021; Hobart and Kneese 2020; Puig de la Bellacasa 2017.

Chapter 1: The Bureaucratic Politics of Good Living

1. Literally, "brother." The term tended to be used in two ways. Sometimes, it was used for Evangelical church members (which would apply here; Herculiano was a Protestant). But it was also often used to refer to movement actors more generally, especially within participatory planning spaces. So, President Morales was often referred to as "el hermano Evo," but also *hermano* was used as a form of address for workshop participants.

2. I have used the real names (rather than pseudonyms) for public figures in leadership roles, including the former Minister of Health and Sports (Nila Heredia) and the former Vice-Minister of Traditional Medicine and Interculturality (Alberto Camaqui).

3. Kate Centellas (forthcoming) has similarly observed that some middle- and upper-class Bolivians with whom she spoke did not believe that Telesalud, the state's virtual satellite-enabled telehealth network, had actually been implemented. She points out that the system had in fact been fully implemented across the country, but people making these claims almost never set foot in public clinics.

4. Nancy Postero (2017) has argued, for instance, that as the MAS sought to translate its official rhetoric into practice, it remained constrained by working within an existing liberal capitalist system. In one of her central examples, she highlights how the new national constitution, enacted in 2009, selectively took up elements of proposals from the *Pacto de Unidad* (Pact of Unity, comprising six major social movements), but fell short of the Pacto's more radical demands. She argues that state-led decolonization took shape primarily in the realm of state rhetoric and public performance that, while also an important site of meaning-making, ultimately reentrenched colonial state power. Similarly, Aymara sociologist Felix Patzi Paco, the first minister of education under Morales from 2006 to 2007, reflected that activist proposals for decolonization were central to elaborating societal models that were "totally distinct from those of liberal capitalism and state socialism" (2014, 7); however, according to

236 NOTES TO CHAPTER 1

him, the Morales administration's engagement with these proposals in realms like education policy were more "symbolic" than concrete.

5. Here, I broadly engage Michel Foucault's (1980; 1990) concept of bio-power as the institutional techniques, mechanisms, and strategies for disciplining bodies and controlling populations that were especially central to the formation of public health and medicine as fields. More specifically, I engage with scholars that have re-theorized biopolitics to examine to operation of colonial state power. These works have emphasized how state policies have often invoked benevolent projects of keeping Indigenous populations physically alive—what Lisa Stevenson (2014) calls "life itself"—while also thieving the very relations and lands that sustain Indigenous lives and well-being (Million 2020; Morgensen 2011). To this end, colonial biopolitics has also often entailed the pathologization of Indigenous bodies, practices, and forms of life-making as threats to biological health in need of intervention and regulation. Biopolitics never work seamlessly—and extensions of state benevolence in the name of saving lives have just as often been paired with state abandonment and neglect (where both care and its withdrawal often work hand-in-hand as strategies of domination).

6. On the 1952 revolution and state-building in its aftermath, see Dunkerley 1984; Gotkowitz 2007; Rivera Cusicanqui 1984; Zavaleta Mercado 2018.

7. See Castellanos 2017; de la Cadena 2000; Stepan 1991; Jarrín 2017; Wade 2010.

8. See Bjork-James 2020, Ellison 2018, Mamani Ramirez 2004, and Farthing and Kohl 2014 for accounts of the uprising in El Alto and the aftermath.

9. Goodale 2019; Gustafson 2009a; Postero 2017; Regalsky 2009; 2010; Schavelzón 2012.

10. Many scholars, critiquing how universalism often reproduces singular, Eurocentric framings, have emphasized pluriversalism as a key component of an anticolonial politics (de la Cadena 2015; Escobar 2020). While Bolivian policymakers have sometimes also emphasized aspects of incorporating multiple worlds into policy, my understanding is that Alonzo included the term "universal" here to specifically refer to universal health care (which the Morales administration was working to establish).

11. Particularly with the rise of left-leaning governments across Latin America at the start of the twenty-first century, political anthropologists have raised questions about how people working for and with the state understand the state to be a vehicle for social transformation, accountable to activist political bases. For Naomi Schiller (2018), activist community media producers in Venezuela understood the state as under construction—and their own participation in state press conferences as "meaningful opportunities for the poor to participate in revolutionary statecraft" (5). In contrast, Kregg Hetherington (2020) suggests that leftist and environmentalist activist bureaucrats

in Paraguay came into office with the hope that they would be able to regulate and transform the soy industry; yet they found their ability to enact change curtailed by the entrenched form of the "soy state."

12. On Latin American Social Medicine, see also Krieger 2003; Waitzkin et al. 2001; Yamada 2003.

13. *Nuestra realidad* was a claim to the specificity of the Bolivian context, one that many also framed in terms of Bolivia's pluricultural and majority Indigenous demographic make-up. As Dr. Yolanda Vargas, a physician who played a central role on the ministry team that developed the SAFCI, reflected in a later essay, "We had to define the principles and the operative mechanism from the standpoint of *nuestra realidad*. This was the great challenge, to respond relevantly to this plurinational reality in a unique political, legal, historical and organizational context" (2013, 56, my translation).

14. Bolivian health reforms were thus an important forerunner to what Vivian Laurens, César Abadía-Barrero, and Mario Hernández (2023) describe as a growing paradigm shift among social medicine activists across the Latin American continent. They write, "Based on the perspective of *Buen Vivir*, Indigenous groups have criticized the dependance of LASM on modernist Western epistemology to shape both its theory and its practice. . . . As a result of these critiques from *Buen Vivir*, in the last decade LASM scholars/activists have engaged more purposefully with this Indigenous epistemology and social movement. The goal has been to open room for other ways of understanding and improving health conditions and to incorporate those lessons to reimagine the work of LASM" (96). Note that in Bolivia the term "Vivir Bien" is more common, while in Ecuador the term "Buen Vivir" took shape. Both mean the same thing ("good living"). As the phrase has traveled to other activist contexts in Latin America, "Buen Vivir" has been the more common iteration.

15. On intercultural health policies in Latin America, see Carreño-Calderón 2021; Guerra-Reyes 2019; Vega 2018.

16. The neighboring countries of Bolivia and Peru share many cultural and geographical similarities, although their national politics have taken different forms. Perhaps that is why Ramón used Peruvian intercultural health policies as a foil for Bolivian ones. However, as I go on to describe in Chapter 3, Bolivian maternal intercultural health programs shared many overlaps with Peruvian policies, as well as with other maternal health policies in the region. Bolivian maternal health programs also ultimately replicated some of the problems Ramón described, as they brought women into the purview of biomedical obstetric care.

17. For a report on the Mi Agua program and potable water supply in Bolivia, see Estado Plurinacional de Bolivia 2021.

18. Anthias 2018; Calla 2020; Gustafson 2020; Postero 2017; Webber 2009.

19. On the Morales administration's health care spending (and its limitations), see Salazar 2020. On global dynamics of neoliberalism and the role of NGOs in the provision of services, see Keshavjee 2014; Gupta and Sharma 2006; Nguyen 2010.

20. On humanitarianism and human rights paradigms, see Bornstein and Redfield 2011; Fassin 2012; Ticktin 2011.

21. Resonantly, anthropologists have also long argued that states are not coherent entities; they are made of often diverse institutions, actors, and projects, including close coordinations with nonstate entities. Yet state can be made to *appear* coherent through work that scholars have variably described as magic, fantasy, or the construction of an "idea" (Abrams 1988; Coronil 1997; Navaro-Yashin 2002).

Chapter 2: Reorienting Care

1. I used the term "unmarked" here and throughout the text to highlight how people may position themselves as the norm, or "just Bolivian."

2. On regimes of mestizaje and racial formation, see de la Cadena 2000; Roberts 2012; Rivera Cusicanqui 1984; 2010; Macusaya Cruz 2020; Molina 2021. For phenotype as an enduring index of race, see Ravindran (2020; 2021).

3. On the complexities of medical paternalism, see Biehl 2007; Roberts 2012; Singer 2022.

4. See Briggs and Mantini Briggs 2003; 2016; Huayhua 2013; Roberts 2012.

5. Other scholars have likewise shown how routinization and practice uphold racial hierarchies. For example, Aisha Beliso-De Jesús (2020) shows how broader structures of white supremacy are sustained through embodied practice. Building from conversations about subject formation in anthropology, she argues that U.S. police academy training relies on an embodied process of "molding" officers into the norms of white supremacy through a focus on deference, militarized uniformity, and athleticism. She suggests that moves to diversify the police force do not challenge these norms; instead, training works to absorb Black and Latinx officers into an unmarked white standard, even as it positions them as always already out-of-place.

6. For more on the ELAM and Cuban medical humanitarianism, see Brotherton 2012; Feinsilver 1993; Huish and Kirk 2007.

7. The doctor's approach to care for Aymara-speaking patients arguably remains embedded in what Jonathan Rosa describes as regimes of modern governance that naturalize the relationship between language, race, and the body, making such assemblages appear inevitable: "Languages are perceived as racially embodied and race is perceived as linguistically intelligible, which results in the overdetermination of racial embodiment and communicative practice" (2019, 2).

Chapter 3: Warm and Cold

1. Medical anthropologists and sociologists have increasingly called for greater attention to the role of men in reproduction, noting the need to understand the specificity and diversity of gender roles mobilized in reproduction (Almeling2020; Inhorn 2020; Inhorn and Wentzell 2011; Wentzell 2013).

2. On sobreparto, see Larme and Leatherman 2003; Loza and Álvarez Quispe 2011; Kuberska 2016.

3. Even as STS and new materialist approaches have increasingly come to pay attention to the agency or vibrancy of matter, they do not always cite or engage long-standing Indigenous theorizations on the subject. See Hokowhitu 2020, TallBear 2017, and Todd 2016 for critiques of these exclusions.

4. See Dominique Behague (2002) and Elizabeth Roberts (2012) on how women in Brazil and Ecuador, respectively, may prefer C-sections because of their associations with privatized, better quality care.

5. Sarah Pinto (2008) argues, for example, in the context of her work in Uttar Pradesh, India, that international agencies' creation of the category of the "traditional midwife" obscured divisions of labor between those who delivered the infant and those who provided postpartum care.

6. For more on the history of traditional birth attendants and skilled birth attendants in Latin America and in global health policy more broadly, see Dixon 2020; El Kotni 2019; Guerra-Reyes 2019; Jordan 1989.

7. Kathryn Gallien (2015) also notes, for example, that some women that she interviewed who assisted in births identified as yatiris, rather than parteras, because they also engaged in ritual healing.

8. On social reproduction, see Federici 2004; S. Ferguson 2016; 2020; Glenn 1992; Meehan and Strauss 2015; Vogel 2013.

Chapter 4: Embodied Redistribution

1. In Bolivia, the umbrella term *medicina tradicional e ancestral* (traditional and ancestral medicine) encompasses a diversity of practitioners who were historically the mainstay of care in many Indigenous and campesino communities. "Traditional and ancestral medicine" is itself a political construct used to classify a range of practices. Although many kinds of healing practice exist in Bolivia—varying by geography, community, and body of knowledge—in this book I engage with two prominent forms of healing in contemporary urbanized Aymara communities: ritual healing (practiced by *yatiris*, *amawt'as*, and *espiritistas*) and natural healing (practiced by *naturistas*). I use the specific term for the healer's specialty when relevant; when speaking in broader terms I use the term "traditional healer" (reflecting the Bolivian political terminology) or simply, "healer."

2. On the professionalization of healing as well as incorporation of biomed-

ical technologies, see Adams 2001; Blaikie 2019; Hampshire and Owusu 2013; Kim 2009; Langwick 2008; 2011.

3. These debates also echoed others, such as once prominent debates between cultural critic and orthodox Marxist approaches to medical anthropology (Morgan 1987).

4. For many scholars working in the Bolivian Andes, expectations that the state should also engage in gifting and redistribution can be linked to long-standing practices of patronage—in which, for example, people might exchange their support for political figures and others in a position of authority in return for jobs, favors, and material support (Albro 2007; Shakow 2011; 2014). Patronage practices have also frequently been a source of local debate and contention—as people (including many Indigenous, campesino, and working-class Bolivians) have also criticized them as running counter to liberal norms of governance or promoting political corruption. Notably, the Morales administration vowed to eliminate patronage as a corrupt practice—and yet, also sometimes invoked similar ethical frames, particularly around its own projects of wealth redistribution. Yet while people sometimes criticized patronage as a corrupt practice, many of them nonetheless also continued to engage with it as a meaningful ethical practice (Shakow 2011). Expectations that the state should redistribute were tied to historically rooted understandings of morally appropriate uses of political authority and how people brought those with more power and resources into relations of gifting and exchange (Winchell 2022).

5. On capitalism as contingent, heterogeneous, and non-totalizing, see also Tsing 2015; Gibson-Graham 1996; 2006.

6. De la Cadena also engages in conversation with Karen Barad's (2007) concept of intra-action, as well as Marilyn Strathern's (2005, 63) distinction between "relations between entities (where entities appear to preexist the relation) and those that bring entities into existence (where entities are through the relation)" (de la Cadena 2015, 102).

7. Indigenous feminist scholars have demonstrated how settler liberal projects treat bodies and lands as separate, autonomous entities—as well as resources that can be plundered. Yet, as they point out, Indigenous theorizations of the intimate connection between body and land—or between human and nonhuman entities—open up possibilities for challenging dominant extractive regimes and collapsing "the settler scale that separates humans, lands, animals, and so on" (Goeman 2017, 101; see also Grande 2021; Yazzie 2018).

8. On ritual healing practice in the Bolivian Andes, see Burman 2017; Canessa 2012; Fernández Juárez 2004.

9. Anthropologists working in other recently urbanizing areas of the Bo-

livian Andes have noted similar dynamics, as Indigenous ritual specialists have expressed concerns about how "city thinking" ruptured relations with a more-than-human community (Alderman 2022) or introduced a new iteration of colonial sickness, a strange spirit (ñanqha) that might infest the body (Burman 2017).

10. Resonantly, Larisa Jašarević (2011; 2017) has argued that studies of medical pluralism often tend to overemphasize the underlying rationalities of healing or approach nonbiomedical healing systems as symbolic representations; she urges use instead to center the ontologically plural ways people embody and experience economic precarity.

11. Abercrombie 1998; Burman 2017; Canessa 2012; Nash 1993; Gordillo 2004; Taussig 2010; Weismantel 2001.

12. Alice Street (2014), writing in the context of Papua New Guinean hospitals, resonantly argues that people engage hospital technologies to make themselves visible as social actors within relations, in the hopes that doing so might also materialize better health outcomes.

13. On how traditional medicine is also used to "fill in gaps" in health care systems in contexts where there are resource shortages, see Brotherton 2012; Hampshire and Owusu 2013; Langwick 2008; Sheehan 2009.

14. In her writing on tribal gaming in the United States, Jessica Cattelino notes that dominant settler discourses position the accumulation of capital as a sign of Indigenous inauthenticity. Pointing to what she calls the "double-bind of need-based sovereignty," she argues, "American Indian tribal nations (like other polities) require economic resources to exercise sovereignty, and their revenues often derive from their governmental rights; however, once they exercise economic power, the legitimacy of tribal sovereignty and citizenship is challenged in law, public culture, and everyday interactions within settler society" (2010, 235–36).

Chapter 5: Doctor, Patient, Kin

1. While Rivera Cusicanqui (1990) positions the ayllu as a counter to liberal formations, see also Mark Goodale (2009) on how ayllu communities have also selectively engaged and reworked liberal legal systems at the local level.

2. On documentation and data collection, particularly in the context of national and global health policies, see Adams 2016; Biruk 2018; Erikson 2018; Pigg, Erikson, and Inglis 2018; Saluk 2022; Suh 2021; Strong 2020.

3. Eve Tuck describes what she calls "damage-centered research" as "research that intends to document peoples' pain and brokenness to hold those in power accountable for their oppression" (2009, 409). She points out that a shortcoming of such research is that it often treats brokenness as inherent to marginalized communities, without sufficiently reckoning with the role of

racism and ongoing colonization in producing damage. Dian Million's (2020) critique of health data collection takes up the concern that this form of research roots anomie in Indigenous communities themselves. And like Tuck, she calls for a greater emphasis on Indigenous desires and life-making projects as a way to move away from damage-centered narratives.

4. These were the instructions given to providers at the time of my research in 2015. However, a more recent set of instructions for the carpetas (Ministerio de Salud y Deportes 2019, 43) also suggests additional ways of drawing relations—for example, for relations in which one person is "dominant" or relations are "intense."

5. As Seda Saluk (2021) has argued, state and global health moves to "datify" care simultaneously mobilize unequal care labor and reentrench existing social hierarchies that render marginalized groups the subject of surveillance.

6. Cal Biruk demonstrates how survey data is always already "cooked" from its design, collection, and implementation. In tracing these processes, Biruk pushes back against the idea that data-collecting fieldworkers are especially prone to fudging data; rather, "it is the creative and innovative tactics of fieldworkers that ensure that data collection proceeds smoothly, and their artful negotiation between top-down standards and bottom-up particularities—a kind of cooking data—that produces clean data as arbitrated by survey research standards" (2018, 8).

7. At the time of this incident, universal health care had not yet been implemented, and public insurance only covered children up to five. Javi was six.

8. Although these accusations of "wanting to take advantage" unfolded within a context of Bolivian political reforms, scholars working in other contexts have likewise highlighted how practices of exchange in the medical setting can be subject to accusations of corruption. Rima Praspaliauskiene (2016) demonstrates, for example, how in postsocialist Slovenia, people frequently gift envelopes of money to doctors. While patients who give these gifts understand them to facilitate care, others have critiqued such practices as a form of bribery.

Chapter 6: Accountable Care

1. In Bolivia and some other Latin American countries, the verb *renegar* is commonly used to mean complain, to denounce, to get angry about something. However, in some other Spanish-speaking countries, *renegar* is not commonly used. The verb *quejarse* (to complain) has a somewhat similar connotation.

2. The "Túpac Kataris" was often the name used as shorthand for the Sole Departmental Federation of Campesino Workers of La Paz Túpac Katari. The

"Bartolinas" were shorthand for the women's agricultural union, the Bartolina Sisa National Confederation of Campesina, Indigenous, and Native Women of Bolivia (*Confederación Nacional de Mujeres Campesinas Indígenas Originarias de Bolivia "Bartolina Sisa"*).

3. The requirement to spend 15.5 percent of the munical government's share of national tax revenue on health care was codified under Law 475 (Asamblea Legislativa Plurinacional de Bolivia 2013b) and recodified under the universal health care Law 1152 (Asamblea Legislativa Plurinacional de Bolivia 2019).

4. Dokumaci 2020; Finch 2022; Hobart and Kneese 2020; Puig de la Bellacasa 2017.

Conclusion: Political Aftermaths

1. See Abimbola and Pai 2020; Affun-Adegbulu and Adegbulu 2020; Büyüm et al. 2020; Jumbam 2020; Krugman 2023; Lawrence and Hirsch 2020; Richardson 2020.

2. See, for example, Rivera Cusicanqui's (1991) discussion of *Pachakuti* as overturning.

REFERENCES

Abadía-Barrero, César. 2022. *Health in Ruins: The Capitalist Destruction of Medical Care at a Colombian Maternity Hospital*. Experimental Futures. Durham, NC: Duke University Press.

Abercrombie, Thomas Alan. 1998. *Pathways of Memory and Power: Ethnography and History Among an Andean People*. Madison: University of Wisconsin Press.

Abimbola, Seye, and Madhukar Pai. 2020. "Will Global Health Survive Its Decolonisation?" *Lancet (London, England)* 396 (10263): 1627–28.

Abrams, Philip. 1988. "Notes on the Difficulty of Studying the State." *Journal of Historical Socioloy* 1 (1): 11–42. https://doi.org/10.1002/9781444309706.ch1.

Adams, Vincanne. 2001. "The Sacred in the Scientific: Ambiguous Practices of Science in Tibetan Medicine." *Cultural Anthropology* 16 (4): 542–75.

———. 2016. *Metrics: What Counts in Global Health*. Critical Global Health—Evidence, Efficacy, Ethnography. Durham, NC: Duke University Press.

Affun-Adegbulu, Clara, and Opemiposi Adegbulu. 2020. "Decolonising Global (Public) Health: From Western Universalism to Global Pluriversalities." *BMJ Global Health* 5 (8):e002947. https://doi.org/10.1136/bmjgh-2020-002947.

Ahmed, Sara. 2006. "The Nonperformativity of Antiracism." *Meridians* 7 (1): 104–26. https://doi.org/10.2979/MER.2006.7.1.104.

———. 2021. *Complaint!* Durham, NC: Duke University Press.

Albó, Xavier. 2009. "Suma Qamaña = El Buen Convivir." *Revista Obets* 4: 25–40.

Albó, Xavier, Godofredo Sandoval, and Tomás Greaves. 1981. *Chukiyawu: La Cara Aymara de La Paz*. Vol. 2. La Paz, Bolivia: Editorial e Imprenta Alenkar.

Albro, Robert. 2007. "Indigenous Politics in Bolivia's Evo Era: Clientelism,

Llunkerío, and the Problem of Stigma." *Urban Anthropology and Studies of Cultural Systems and World Economic Development* 36 (3): 281–320.

———. 2010. "Counfounding Cultural Citizenship and Constitutional Reform in Bolivia." *Latin American Perspectives* 37 (3): 71–90.

Alderman, Jonathan. 2020. "Bolivia Under Covid-19: The Interim Government and Autonomous Responses." November 6, 2020. https://calacs.wp.st-an drews.ac.uk/2020/11/06/bolivia-under-covid-19-the-interim-government -and-autonomous-responses-by-jonathan-alderman/.

———. 2022. "'City Thinking': Rural Urbanisation and Mobility in Andean Bolivia." *Bulletin of Latin American Research* 41 (1): 21–36. https://doi.org/10.1111 /blar.13214.

Allen, Catherine J. 2002. *The Hold Life Has: Coca and Cultural Identity in an Andean Community*. 2nd. ed. Washington, DC: Smithsonian Institution Press.

Almeling, Rene. 2020. *Guynecology: The Missing Science of Men's Reproductive Health*. Oakland: University of California Press.

Álvarez Quispe, Walter, and Carmen Beatriz Loza. 2014. "Medicinas Tradicionales Andinas y Su Despenalización: Entrevista Con Walter Álvarez Quispe." *História, Ciências, Saúde-Manguinhos* 21 (4): 1475–86. https://doi.org/10.1590/ S0104-59702014000400012.

Amrute, Sareeta. 2016. *Encoding Race, Encoding Class: Indian IT Workers in Berlin*. https://doi.org/10.1215/9780822374275.

Andaya, Elise. 2014. *Conceiving Cuba : Reproduction, Women, and the State in the Post-Soviet Era*. New Brunswick, NJ: Rutgers University Press.

Anria, Santiago. 2018. *When Movements Become Parties: The Bolivian MAS in Comparative Perspective*. Cambridge, UK: Cambridge University Press.

Anthias, Penelope. 2018. *Limits to Decolonization: Indigeneity, Territory, and Hydrocarbon Politics in the Bolivian Chaco*. Ithaca, NY: Cornell University Press.

Arigho-Stiles, Olivia. 2024. "Landscapes of Struggle: Katarista Perspectives on the Environment in Bolivia, 1960–1990." In *Land Back: Relational Landscapes of Indigenous Resistance Across the Americas*, ed. Heather Dorries and Michelle Daigle, 39–59. Washington, DC: Dumbarton Oaks.

Arnold, Denise, and Juan de Dios Yapita. 2002. *Las Wawas Del Inka: Hacia La Salud Materna Intercultural En Algunas Comunidades Andinas*. La Paz, Bolivia: Instituto de Lengua y Cultura Aymara (ILCA).

Arvin, Maile. 2019. *Possessing Polynesians: The Science of Settler Colonial Whiteness in Hawaii and Oceania*. Durham, NC: Duke University Press.

Asamblea Legislativa Plurinacional de Bolivia. 2013a. "Ley N° 459: Ley de Medicina Tradicional Ancestral Boliviana."

———. 2013b. "Ley N° 475: Ley de Prestaciones Servicios de Salud Integral Del Estado Plurinacional de Bolivia."

————. 2019. " Ley N° 1152: Ley Modificatoria a La Ley N° 475 De30 de Diciembre de 2013, de Prestaciones de Servicios de Salud Integral Del Estado Plurinacional de Bolivia, Modificada Por Ley No 1069 de 28 de Mayo de 2018. 'Hacia El Sistema Único de Salud, Universal y Gratuito'".

Aulino, Felicity. 2019. *Rituals of Care: Karmic Politics in an Aging Thailand.* Ithaca, NY: Cornell University Press.

Babis, Deby. 2014. "The Role of Civil Society Organizations in the Institutionalization of Indigenous Medicine in Bolivia." *Social Science & Medicine* 123 (December): 287–94. https://doi.org/10.1016/j.socscimed.2014.07.034.

————. 2018. "Exploring the Emergence of Traditional Healer Organizations: The Case of an Ethno-Medical Association in Bolivia." *Health Sociology Review* 27 (2): 136–52. https://doi.org/10.1080/14461242.2018.1452624.

Bailey, Jennifer L., and Torbjørn L. Knutsen. 1987. "Surgery Without Anaesthesia: Bolivia's Response to Economic Chaos." *The World Today* 43 (3): 47–51.

Bajaj, Simar Singh, Lwando Maki, and Fatima Cody Stanford. 2022. "Vaccine Apartheid: Global Cooperation and Equity." *The Lancet* 399 (10334): 1452–53. https://doi.org/10.1016/S0140-6736(22)00328-2.

Barad, Karen. 2003. "Posthumanist Performativity: Toward an Understanding of How Matter Comes to Matter." *Signs: Journal of Women in Culture and Society* 28 (3).

————. 2007. *Meeting the Universe Halfway: Quantum Physics and the Entanglement of Matter and Meaning.* Durham, NC: Duke University Press. https://doi.org/10.1515/9780822388128.

Barragán, Rossana. 2011. "The Census and the Making of a Social 'Order' in Nineteenth-Century Bolivia." In *Histories of Race and Racism: The Andes and Mesoamerica from Colonial Times to the Present,* ed. Laura Gotkowitz. Durham, NC: Duke University Press.

Bastien, Joseph W. 1990. "Community Health Workers in Bolivia: Adapting to Traditional Roles in the Andean Community." *Social Science & Medicine* 30 (3): 281–87.

Bates, Victoria. 2018. "'Humanizing' Healthcare Environments: Architecture, Art and Design in Modern Hospitals." *Design for Health* 2 (1): 5–19.

Bear, Laura, Karen Ho, Anna Tsing, and Sylvia Yanagisako. 2015. "Gens: A Feminist Manifesto for the Study of Capitalism." *Cultural Anthropology* 30.

Béhague, Dominique. 2002. "Beyond the Simple Economics of Cesarean Section Birthing: Women's Resistance to Social Inequality." *Culture, Medicine and Psychiatry* 26: 473–507.

Beliso-De Jesús, Aisha M. 2020. "The Jungle Academy: Molding White Supremacy in American Police Recruits." *American Anthropologist* 122 (1): 143–56.

Bennet, Jane. 2010. *Vibrant Matter: A Political Ecology of Things.* Durham, NC: Duke University Press.

Bernstein, Alissa. 2013. "Transformative Medical Education and the Making of New Clinical Subjectivities Through Cuban-Bolivian Medical Diplomacy." In *Health Travels: Cuban Health (Care) On and Off the Island,* ed. Nancy Burke, 154–77. San Francisco: University of California Medical Humanities Press.

——. 2017. "Personal and Political Histories in the Designing of Health Reform Policy in Bolivia." *Social Science & Medicine* 177 (March): 231–38. https://doi.org/10.1016/j.socscimed.2017.01.028.

——. 2018. "Proliferating Policy: Technologies, Performance, and Aesthetics in the Circulation and Governance of Health Care Reform in Bolivia." *PoLAR: Political and Legal Anthropology Review,* 41 (2): 262–76.

Berry, Nicole. 2010. *Unsafe Motherhood: Mayan Maternal Mortality and Subjectivity in Post-War Guatemala.* New York and Oxford, UK: Berghahn Books.

Biehl, Joao. 2007. *Will to Live: AIDS Therapies and the Politics of Survival.* Princeton, NJ: Princeton University Press.

Biruk, Crystal. 2018. *Cooking Data: Culture and Politics in an African Research World.* Durham, NC: Duke University Press.

Bjork-James, Carwil. 2020. *The Sovereign Street: Making Revolution in Urban Bolivia.* Tucson, AZ: University of Arizona Press.

Black, Steven P. 2018. "The Ethics and Aesthetics of Care." *Annual Review of Anthropology* 47: 79–95.

Blaikie, Calum. 2019. "Mainstreaming Marginality: Traditional Medicine and Primary Healthcare in Himalayan India." *Asian Medicine* 14 (1): 145–72. https://doi.org/10.1163/15734218-12341438.

Blaser, Mario. 2009. "Political Ontology: Cultural Studies Without 'Cultures'?" *Cultural Studies* 23 (5–6): 873–96.

Bohrt, Marcelo A. 2019. "Racial Ideologies, State Bureaucracy, and Decolonization in Bolivia." *Bolivian Studies Journal* 25: 7–28.

Booth, Amy. 2020. "Bolivia's New Health Minister Promises Universal Health Care." *The Lancet* 396 (10266): 1872.

Bornstein, Erica, and Peter Redfield, eds. 2011. *Forces of Compassion.* Santa Fe, NM: SAR PRESS.

Bridges, Khiara. 2011. *Reproducing Race: An Ethnography of Pregnancy as a Site of Racialization.* Berkeley and Los Angeles: University of California Press.

Briggs, Charles, and Clara Mantini-Briggs. 2003. *Stories in the Time of Cholera: Racial Profiling During a Medical Nightmare.* Berkeley, CA: University of California Press.

——. 2016. *Tell Me Why My Children Died: Rabies, Indigenous Knowledge, and Communicative Justice.* Durham, NC, and London: Duke University Press.

Brodwin, Paul. 2013. *Everyday Ethics: Voices from the Front Line of Community Psychiatry.* Oakland: University of California Press.

Brotherton, Pierre Sean. 2012. *Revolutionary Medicine: Health and the Body in Post-Soviet Cuba*. Durham, NC: Duke University Press.

Buch, Elana. 2018. *Inequalities of Aging: Paradoxes of Independence in American Home Care*. New York: New York University Press.

Burman, Anders. 2012. "Places to Think With, Books to Think About: Words, Experience and the Decolonization of Knowledge in the Bolivian Andes." *Human Architecture: Journal of the Sociology of Self Knowledge* X (1): 101–20.

———. 2017. *Indigeneity and Decolonization in the Bolivian Andes: Ritual Practice and Activism*. Lanham, MD: Lexington Books.

Büyüm, Ali Murad, Cordelia Kenney, Andrea Koris, Laura Mkumba, and Yadurshini Raveendran. 2020. "Decolonising Global Health: If Not Now, When?" *BMJ Global Health* 5 (8): e003394. https://doi.org/10.1136/bmjgh-2020-003394.

Calla, Pamela. 2020. "The Difficulties of Connecting Anti-Extractivist and Anti-Racist Struggles in Contemporary Bolivia." In *Black and Indigenous Resistance in the Americas: From Multiculturalism to Racist Backlash*, ed. Juliet Hooker, 189–215. Lanham, MD: Lexington Books.

Cameron, John D. 2009a. "Hacia La Alcaldia: The Municipalization of Peasant Politics in the Andes." *Latin American Perspectives* 36 (4): 64–82. https://doi.org/10.1177/0094582X09338586.

———. 2009b. "'Development Is a Bag of Cement': The Infrapolitics of Participatory Budgeting in the Andes." *Development in Practice* 19 (6): 692–701. https://doi.org/10.1080/09614520903026835.

Campos Navarro, Roberto. 1997. "Curanderismo, Medicina Indígena y Proceso de Legalización." *Nueva Antropología* 16 (53): 67–87.

Campos Navarro, Roberto, Fabiola García Vargas, Uzziel Barrón, Mariana Salazar, and Javier Cabral Soto. 1997. "La Satisfacción Del Enfermo Hospitalizado: Empleo de Hamacas En Un Hospital Rural Del Sureste de México." *Revista Médica IMSS* 35 (4): 265–72.

Canessa, Andrew. 2012. *Intimate Indigeneities: Race, Sex, and History in the Small Spaces of Andean Life. Narrating Native Histories*. Durham, NC: Duke University Press.

Carreño-Calderón, Alejandra. 2021. "Living Well and Health Practices Among Aymara People in Northern Chile." *Latin American Perspectives* 48 (3): 69–81.

Castellanos, M. Bianet. 2017. "Introduction: Settler Colonialism in Latin America." *American Quarterly* 69 (4): 777–81.

———. 2021. *Indigenous Dispossession: Housing and Maya Indebtedness in Mexico*. Stanford, CA: Stanford University Press.

Castro-Gómez, Santiago. 2005. *La Poscolonialidad Explicada a Los Niños*. Editorial Universidad del Cauca; Instituto Pensar, Universidad Javeriana.

Cattelino, Jessica R. 2010. "The Double-Bind of American Need-Based Sover-

eignty." *Cultural Anthropology* 25 (2): 235–62. https://doi.org/10.1111/j.1548
-1360.2010.01058.x.

Centellas, Kate M. Forthcoming. "Satellites and Skepticism: Decolonial Technocratic Tensions in Bolivia."

Centro de Documentación e Información Bolivia (CEDIB). 2013. "Indígenas: Quién Gana, Quién Pierde: Datos Comparativos de La Población Indígena, Censos de Población, 2001 y 2012." CEDIB. http://www.cedib.org/wp-content/ uploads/2013/08/Tabla-Poblacion-Indigena1.pdf.

Chatterjee, Piya. 2001. *A Time for Tea: Women, Labor, and Post/Colonial Politics on an Indian Plantation*. Durham, NC: Duke University Press.

Choque, María Eugenia, and Carlos Mamani. 2001. "Reconstitucion Del Ayllu y Derechos de Los Pueblos Indigenas: El Movimiento Indio En Los Andes de Bolivia." *Journal of Latin American Anthropology* 6 (1): 202–24.

Choque Canqui, Roberto. 2010. "El Manifesto de Tiwanaku (1973) y El Inicio de La Descolonización." *Fuentes. Revista de La Biblioteca y Archivo Histórico de La Asamblea Legislativa Plurinacional* 4 (11): 11–15.

Choquehuanca, David. 2010. "Hacia La Reconstruccion Del Vivir Bien." *America Latina En Movimiento* 452: 8–13.

Claros, Luis. 2022. "A modo de presentación: momentos de la crisis." In *Crisis política en Bolivia 2019–2020*, ed. Luis Claros and Vladimir Díaz Cuellar, 7–17. La Paz, Bolivia: Plural Editores.

Conaghan, Catherine M., James M. Malloy, and Luis A. Abugattas. 1990. "Business and the Boys": The Politics of Neoliberalism in the Central Andes." *Latin American Research Review* 25 (2): 3–30.

Cooke, Bill, and Uma Kothari, eds. 2001. *Participation: The New Tyranny?* London; New York: Zed Books.

Cooper, Amy. 2019. *State of Health: Pleasure and Politics in Venezuelan Health Care Under Chávez*. Oakland: University of California Press.

Cordoba, Diana, and Kees Jansen. 2016. "Realigning the Political and the Technical: NGOs and the Politicization of Agrarian Development in Bolivia." *The European Journal of Development Research* 28 (3): 447–64.

Coronil, Fernando. 1997. *The Magical State: Nature, Money, and Modernity in Venezuela*. Chicago: University of Chicago Press.

Coulthard, Glen Sean. 2014. *Red Skin, White Masks: Rejecting the Colonial Politics of Recognition*. Minneapolis: University of Minnesota Press. http://dx.doi.org/10.5749/minnesota/9780816679645.001.0001.

Crandon-Malamud, Libbet. 1991. *From the Fat of Our Souls: Social Change, Political Process, and Medical Pluralism in Bolivia*. Berkeley: University of California Press.

Dangl, Benjamin. 2019. *The Five Hundred Year Rebellion: Indigenous Movements and the Decolonization of History in Bolivia*. Chico, CA: AK Press.

Davis, Dana-Aín. 2019. *Reproductive Injustice: Racism, Pregnancy, and Premature Birth*. New York: New York University Press.

Davis-Floyd, Robbie. 1992. *Birth as an American Rite of Passage*. Berkeley: University of California Press.

de la Cadena, Marisol. 2000. *Indigenous Mestizos: The Politics of Race and Culture in Cuzco, Peru, 1919–1991*. Latin America Otherwise. Durham, NC: Duke University Press.

———. 2010. "Indigenous Cosmopolitics in the Andes: Conceptual Reflections Beyond 'Politics.'" *Cultural Anthropology* 25 (2): 334–70. https://doi.org/10.1111/j.1548-1360.2010.01061.x.

———. 2015. *Earth Beings: Ecologies of Practice Across Andean Worlds*. The Lewis Henry Morgan Lectures. Durham, NC: Duke University Press.

Díaz Cuellar, Vladimir. 2022. "Un giro de casi 360 grados: el régimen de noviembre y el retorno del MAS." In *Crisis política en Bolivia 2019–2020*, ed. Luis Claros and Vladimir Díaz Cuellar, 7–17. La Paz, Bolivia: Plural Editores.

Dixon, Lydia Zacher. 2020. *Delivering Health: Midwifery and Development in Mexico*. Policy to Practice. Nashville: Vanderbilt University Press.

Dokumaci, Arseli. 2020. "People as Affordances: Building Disability Worlds Through Care Intimacy." *Current Anthropology* 61 (S21): S97–108. https://doi.org/10.1086/705783.

Dunkerley, James. 1984. *Rebellion in the Veins: Political Struggle in Bolivia, 1952–82*. London: Verso.

EFE. 2023. "Bolivia levanta la emergencia sanitaria por la covid e ingresa a la alerta epidemiológica." SWI swissinfo.ch. July 31, 2023. https://www.swissinfo.ch/spa/coronavirus-bolivia_bolivia-levanta-la-emergencia-sanitaria-por-la-covid-e-ingresa-a-la-alerta-epidemiol%C3%B3gica/48703108.

El Kotni, Mounia. 2019. "Regulating Traditional Mexican Midwifery: Practices of Control, Strategies of Resistance." *Medical Anthropology* 38 (2): 137–51. https://doi.org/10.1080/01459740.2018.1539974.

Ellison, Susan Helen. 2018. *Domesticating Democracy: The Politics of Conflict Resolution in Bolivia*. Durham, NC: Duke University Press.

———. 2023. "We Move Up Levels Together: Dignity, Transformative Marketing, and the Repurposing of Racial Capitalism." *Anthropologica* 65 (2): 1–26.

Erikson, Susan L. 2018. "Cell Phones ≠ Self and Other Problems with Big Data Detection and Containment During Epidemics." *Medical Anthropology Quarterly* 32 (3): 315–39. https://doi.org/10.1111/maq.12440.

Escobar, Arturo. 2004. "Beyond the Third World: Imperial Globality, Global Coloniality and Anti-Globalisation Social Movements." *Third World Quarterly* 25 (1): 207–30.

———. 2020. *Pluriversal Politics*. Durham, NC: Duke University Press.

Espinosa Miñoso, Yuderkys. 2022. *De Por Qué Es Necesario Un Feminismo Descolonial*. Barcelona, Spain: Icaria Editorial.

Estado Plurinacional de Bolivia. 2021. "Informe Nacional Voluntario de Bolivia 2021."

Ewig, Christina. 2010. *Second-Wave Neoliberalism: Gender, Race, and Health Sector Reform in Peru*. University Park: Pennsylvania State University Press.

Fabricant, Nicole. 2009. "Performative Politics: The Camba Countermovement in Eastern Bolivia." *American Ethnologist* 36 (4): 768–83.

Farthing, Linda C., and Thomas Becker. 2021. *Coup: A Story of Violence and Resistance in Bolivia*. Chicago: Haymarket Books.

Farthing, Linda C., and Benjamin H. Kohl. 2014. *Evo's Bolivia: Continuity and Change*. Austin: University of Texas Press.

Farthing, Linda C., and Nancy Romer. 2019. "Urban Gardens Are Blossoming Throughout Bolivia." *City Farmer News*. https://cityfarmer.info/bolivia-community-gardens-in-three-cities-cochabamba-sucre-and-el-alto/.

Fassin, Didier. 2012. *Humanitarian Reason: A Moral History of the Present*. Berkeley: University of California Press.

Federici, Silvia. 2004. *Caliban and the Witch: Women, the Body and Primitive Accumulation*. Brooklyn, NY: Autonomedia.

Feinsilver, Julie. 1993. *Healing the Masses: Cuban Health Politics at Home and Abroad*. Berkeley: University of California Press.

Ferguson, James. 2015. *Give a Man a Fish: Reflections on the New Politics of Distribution*. Durham, NC: Duke University Press.

Ferguson, James, and Tania Li. 2018. "Beyond the 'Proper Job:' Political-Economic Analysis After the Century of Labouring Man." *Working Paper 51*. Cape Town: PLAAS, University of the Western Cape.

Ferguson, Susan. 2016. "Intersectionality and Social-Reproduction Feminisms." *Historical Materialism* 24 (2): 38–60. https://doi.org/10.1163/1569206X-12341471.

———. 2020. *Women and Work: Feminism, Labour, and Social Reproduction*. London: Pluto Press.

Fernández Juárez, Gerardo. 2004. *Yatiris y Chámakanis Del Altiplano Aymara: Sueños, Testimonios y Prácticas Ceremoniales*. 1a. ed. Quito, Ecuador: Abya Yala.

Field, Thomas C. 2014. *From Development to Dictatorship: Bolivia and the Alliance for Progress in the Kennedy Era*. Ithaca, NY: Cornell University Press.

Finch, Aisha K. 2022. "Introduction: Black Feminism and the Practice of Care." *Palimpsest: A Journal on Women, Gender, and the Black International* 11 (1): 1–41. https://doi.org/10.1353/pal.2022.0000.

Foley, Ellen E. 2010. *Your Pocket Is What Cures You: The Politics of Health in Senegal*. New Brunswick, NJ: Rutgers University Press. http://search.ebscohost

.com/login.aspx?direct=true&scope=site&db=nlebk&db=nlabk&AN=321667.

Foronda, Mauricio, and UDAPE. 2023. "COVID-19 en Bolivia: Muertes y Exceso." BoliGráfica. https://www.boligrafica.com/covid-muertes.

Foucault, Michel. 1980. "The Politics of Health in the Eighteenth Century." In *Power/Knowledge: Selected Interviews and Other Writings, 1972–1977*, 166–82. New York: Pantheon.

———. 1990. *The History of Sexuality: Volume 1, An Introduction*. New York: Vintage.

———. 1994. *The Birth of the Clinic : An Archaeology of Medical Perception*. New York: Vintage.

Fraser, Nancy, and Axel Honneth. 2003. *Redistribution or Recognition? A Political-Philosophical Exchange*. Trans. Joel Golb, James Ingram, and Christiane Wilke. London: Verso.

Gallien, Kathryn N. 2015. "Delivering the Nation, Raising the State: Gender, Childbirth and the 'Indian Problem' in Bolivia's Obstetric Movement, 1900–1982." PhD diss. University of Arizona.

Garcia, Angela. 2010. *The Pastoral Clinic: Addiction and Dispossession Along the Rio Grande*. Berkeley: University of California Press.

García Linera, Álvaro, Raquel Gutierrez, Raul Prada, and Luis Tapia. 1999. *El Fantasma Insomne: Pensando El Presente Desde El Manifiesto Comunista*. La Paz, Bolivia: Muela del Diablo Editores.

García Linera, Álvaro, Luis Tapia, Oscar Vega, and Raúl Prada. 2010. *El Estado: Campo de La Lucha*. La Paz, Bolivia: Muela del Diablo Editores.

García, María Elena. 2005. *Making Indigenous Citizens: Identities, Education, and Multicultural Development in Peru*. Stanford, CA: Stanford University Press.

Geidel, Molly. 2010. "'Sowing Death in Our Women's Wombs': Modernization and Indigenous Nationalism in the 1960s Peace Corps and Jorge Sanjinés Yawar Mallku." *American Quarterly* 62 (3): 763–86.

Gibson-Graham, J. K. 1996. *The End of Capitalism (as We Knew It): A Feminist Critique of Political Economy*. Cambridge, MA: Blackwell.

———. 2006. *A Postcapitalist Politics*. Minneapolis: University of Minnesota Press.

Gill, Lesley. 2000. *Teetering on the Rim: Global Restructuring, Daily Life, and the Armed Retreat of the Bolivian State*. New York: Columbia University Press.

Giordano, Cristiana. 2014. *Migrants in Translation: Caring and the Logics of Difference in Contemporary Italy*. Berkeley: University of California Press.

Glenn, Evelyn Nakano. 1992. "From Servitude to Service Work: Historical Continuities in the Racial Division of Paid Reproductive Labor." *Signs: Journal of Women in Culture and Society* 18 (1): 1–43. https://doi.org/10.1086/494777.

Goeman, Mishuana. 2015. "Land as Life: Unsettling the Logics of Containment." In *Native Studies Keywords,* ed. Stephanie Nohelani Teves, Andrea Smith, and Michelle H. Raheja, 71–89. Tucson: University of Arizona Press. https://doi.org/10.2307/j.ctt183gxzb.

———. 2017. "Ongoing Storms and Struggles: Gendered Violence and Resource Exploitation." In *Critically Sovereign: Indigenous Gender, Sexuality, and Feminist Studies,* ed. Joanne Barker, 99–126. Durham, NC: Duke University Press. https://doi.org/10.1215/9780822373162.

González Casanovas, Pedro. 1965. "Internal Colonialism and National Development." *Studies in Comparative International Development* 1 (4): 27–37.

Good, Byron, and Mary-Jo DelVecchio Good. 1993. "Learning Medicine: The Construction of Medical Knowledge at Harvard Medical School." In *Knowledge, Power, and Practice: The Anthropology of Medicine and Everyday Life,* ed. Shirley Lindenbaum and Margaret Lock, 81–107. Berkeley: University of California Press.

Goodale, Mark. 2009. *Dilemmas of Modernity: Bolivian Encounters with Law and Liberalism.* Stanford, CA: Stanford University Press.

———. 2019. *A Revolution in Fragments: Traversing Scales of Justice, Ideology, and Practice in Bolivia.* Durham, NC: Duke University Press.

Goodale, Mark, and Nancy Postero, eds. 2013. *Neoliberalism, Interrupted: Social Change and Contested Governance in Contemporary Latin America.* Stanford, CA: Stanford University Press.

Gordillo, Gastón. 2004. *Landscapes of Devils: Tensions of Place and Memory in the Argentinean Chaco.* Durham, NC: Duke University Press.

Gotkowitz, Laura. 2007. *A Revolution for Our Rights: Indigenous Struggles for Land and Justice in Bolivia, 1880–1952.* Durham, NC: Duke University Press.

Grande, Sandy. 2021. "Care." In *Keywords for Gender and Sexuality Studies,* ed. The Keywords Feminist Editorial Collective, 43–46. New York: New York University Press.

Grisaffi, Thomas. 2019. *Coca Yes, Cocaine No: How Bolivia's Coca Growers Reshaped Democracy.* Durham, NC, and London: Duke University Press.

Guerra-Reyes, Lucia. 2019. *Changing Birth in the Andes: Culture, Policy, and Safe Motherhood in Peru.* Nashville: Vanderbilt University Press.

Gupta, Akhil. 2012. *Red Tape: Bureaucracy, Structural Violence, and Poverty in India.* Durham, NC: Duke University Press.

Gupta, Akhil, and Aradhana Sharma. 2006. "Globalization and Postcolonial States." *Current Anthropology* 27 (2): 277–307.

Gustafson, Bret. 2009a. "Manipulating Cartographies: Plurinationalism, Autonomy, and Indigenous Resurgence in Bolivia." *Anthropology Quarterly* 82 (4): 985–1016.

———. 2009b. *New Languages of the State: Indigenous Resurgence and the Politics of Knowledge in Bolivia.* Durham, NC: Duke University Press.

———. 2020. *Bolivia in the Age of Gas*. Durham, NC: Duke University Press.

———. 2021. "Bolivia's Double Pandemic: A Coup and COVID-19." *Current History* 120 (823): 50–56.

Hall, Stuart. 1996. "When Was the 'Post-Colonial'? Thinking at the Limit." In *The Post-Colonial Question: Common Skies, Divided Horizons*, ed. Iain Chambers and Linda Curti. New York: Routledge.

Hampshire, Kate R., and Samuel Asiedu Owusu. 2013. "Grandfathers, Google, and Dreams: Medical Pluralism, Globalization, and New Healing Encounters in Ghana." *Medical Anthropology* 32 (3): 247–65.

Han, Clara. 2012. *Life in Debt: Times of Care and Violence in Neoliberal Chile*. Berkeley: University of California Press.

Hardin, Jessica A. 2018. *Faith and the Pursuit of Health: Cardiometabolic Disorders in Samoa*. Medical Anthropology. New Brunswick, NJ: Rutgers University Press.

Herrick, Clare, and Kirsten Bell. 2022. "Epidemic Confusions: On Irony and Decolonisation in Global Health." *Global Public Health* 17 (8): 1467–78. https://doi.org/10.1080/17441692.2021.1955400.

Herzfeld, Michael. 1993. *The Social Production of Indifference: Exploring the Symbolic Roots of Western Bureaucracy*. Chicago: University of Chicago Press.

Hetherington, Kregg. 2020. *The Government of Beans: Regulating Life in the Age of Monocrops*. Durham, NC: Duke University Press.

Hobart, Hiʻilei Julia Kawehipuaakahaopulani, and Tamara Kneese. 2020. "Radical Care: Survival Strategies for Uncertain Times." *Social Text* 38 (1 (142)): 1–16.

Hokowhitu, Brendan. 2020. "The Emperor's 'New' Materialisms." In *Routledge Handbook of Critical Indigenous Studies*, ed. Brendan Hokowhitu, Aileen Moreton-Robinson, Linda Tuhiwai-Smith, Chris Andersen, and Steve Larkin, 131–46. Abingdon, Oxon, UK, and New York: Routledge.

Hossain, Naomi. 2010. "Rude Accountability: Informal Pressures on Frontline Bureaucrats in Bangladesh." *Development and Change* 41 (5): 907–28. https://doi.org/10.1111/j.1467-7660.2010.01663.x.

Huanacuni, Fernando. 2010. *Vivir Bien / Buen Vivir : Filosofía, Políticas, Estrategias y Experiencias Regionales*. 1. La Paz, Bolivia: Convenio Andrés Bello: Instituto Internacional de Integración.

Huayhua, Margarita. 2013. "Everyday Discrimination in the Southern Andes." In *Para Quê Serve o Conhecimento Se Eu Não Posso Dividi-Lo? Was Nützt Alles Wissen, Wenn Man Es Nicht Teilen Kann? Gedenkschrift Für Erwin Heinrich Frank*, ed. Birgit Krekeler, Eva König, Stefan Neumann, and Hans-Dieter Ölschleger, 49–58. Berlin, Germany: Ibero-Amerikanisches Institut.

Huish, R., and J. M. Kirk. 2007. "Cuban Medical Internationalism and the Development of the Latin American School of Medicine." *Latin American Perspectives* 34 (6): 77–92.

Hummel, Calla. 2021. *Why Informal Workers Organize: Contentious Politics, Enforcement, and the State*. Oxford. UK: Oxford University Press.

Immerwahr, Daniel. 2015. *Thinking Small: The United States and the Lure of Community Development*. Cambridge, MA: Harvard University Press.

Inhorn, Marcia C. 2020. "Reproducing Men in the Twenty-First Century: Emergent Masculinities, Subjectivities, Biosocialities, and Technologies." *NORMA* 15 (3–4): 299–305. https://doi.org/10.1080/18902138.2020.1831157.

Inhorn, Marcia C., and Emily A. Wentzell. 2011. "Embodying Emergent Masculinities: Men Engaging with Reproductive and Sexual Health Technologies in the Middle East and Mexico." *American Ethnologist* 38 (4): 801–15.

Instituto Nacional de Estadística (INE). 2001. "Censo Nacional de Población y Vivienda."

———. 2012. "Censo Nacional de Población y Vivienda."

Jackson, Shona N. 2012. *Creole Indigeneity: Between Myth and Nation in the Caribbean*. Minneapolis: University of Minnesota Press. https://doi.org/10.5749/minnesota/9780816677757.001.0001.

Janes, Craig R. 1999. "The Health Transition, Global Modernity and the Crisis of Traditional Medicine: The Tibetan Case." *Social Science and Medicine* 48: 1803–20.

Jarrín, Alvaro. 2017. *The Biopolitics of Beauty: Cosmetic Citizenship and Affective Capital in Brazil*. Oakland: University of California Press.

Jašarević, Larisa. 2011. "Lucid Dreaming: Revisiting Medical Pluralism in Postsocialist Bosnia." *Anthropology of East Europe Review* 29 (1): 109–26.

———. 2017. *Health and Wealth on the Bosnian Market: Intimate Debt*. Bloomington: Indiana University Press.

Jensen, Anpotowin, and Victor A. Lopez-Carmen. 2022. "The 'Elephants in the Room' in U.S. Global Health: Indigenous Nations and White Settler Colonialism." *PLOS Global Public Health* 2 (7): e0000719. https://doi.org/10.1371/journal.pgph.0000719.

Johnson, Brian B. 2010. "Decolonization and Its Paradoxes: The (Re)Envisioning of Health Policy in Bolivia." *Latin American Perspectives* 37 (3): 139–59. https://doi.org/10.1177/0094582X10366535.

Jones, Alison, and Kuni Jenkins. 2008. "Rethinking Collaboration: Working the Indigene-Colonizer Hyphen." In *Handbook of Critical and Indigenous Methodologies*, ed. Norman K. Denzin, Yvonna S. Lincoln, and Linda Tuhiwai Smith, 471–86. Thousand Oaks, CA: SAGE.

Jordan, Brigitte. 1989. "Cosmopolitical Obstetrics: Some Insights from the Training of Traditional Midwives." *Social Science & Medicine* 28 (9): 925–37. https://doi.org/10.1016/0277-9536(89)90317-1.

Jumbam, Desmond T. 2020. "How (Not) to Write About Global Health." *BMJ Global Health* 5 (7): e003164. https://doi.org/10.1136/bmjgh-2020-003164.

Kauanui, J. Kēhaulani. 2018. *Paradoxes of Hawaiian Sovereignty: Land, Sex, and the Colonial Politics of State Nationalism*. Durham, NC: Duke University Press.

Kelty, Christopher M. 2017. "Too Much Democracy in All the Wrong Places: Toward a Grammar of Participation." *Current Anthropology* 58 (S15): S77–90. https://doi.org/10.1086/688705.

Keshavjee, Salmaan. 2014. *Blind Spot: How Neoliberalism Infiltrated Global Health*. Vol. 30. Oakland: University of California Press.

Kim, Jongyoung. 2009. "Transcultural Medicine: A Multi-Sited Ethnography on the Scientific-Industrial Networking of Korean Medicine." *Medical Anthropology* 28 (1): 31–64.

Kimball, Natalie L. 2020. *An Open Secret: The History of Unwanted Pregnancy and Abortion in Modern Bolivia*. New Brunswick, NJ: Rutgers University Press.

Klein, Herbert S. 2011. *A Concise History of Bolivia*. 2nd ed. Cambridge Concise Histories. New York: Cambridge University Press.

Kleinman, Arthur. 2007. *What Really Matters: Living a Moral Life Amidst Uncertainty and Danger*. Oxford, UK: Oxford University Press.

——. 2011. "The Divided Self, Hidden Values, and Moral Sensibility in Medicine." *The Lancet* 377 (9768): 804–5.

Klor de Alva, Jorge. 1992. "Colonialism and Postcolonialism as (Latin) American Mirages." *Colonial Latin American Review* 1 (1–2): 3–23. https://doi.org/10.1080/10609169208569787.

Kohl, Benjamin, and Linda C. Farthing. 2006. *Impasse in Bolivia: Neoliberal Hegemony and Popular Resistance*. London: Zed Books.

Koss-Chioino, Joan, Thomas L. Leatherman, and Christine Greenway, eds. 2003. *Medical Pluralism in the Andes*. Theory and Practice in Medical Anthropology and International Health. London; New York: Routledge.

Krieger, Nancy. 2003. "Latin American Social Medicine: The Quest for Social Justice and Public Health." *American Journal of Public Health* 93 (12): 1989–91.

Krugman, Daniel W. 2023. "Global Health and the Elite Capture of Decolonization: On Reformism and the Possibilities of Alternate Paths." Ed. Catherine Kyobutungi. *PLOS Global Public Health* 3 (6): e0002103. https://doi.org/10.1371/journal.pgph.0002103.

Kuberska, Karolina. 2016. "Sobreparto and the Lonely Childbirth: Postpartum Illness and Embodiment of Emotions Among Andean Migrants in Santa Cruz de La Sierra, Bolivia." *Etnografia. Praktyki, Teorie, Doświadczenia*, no. 2, 47–71.

Kukutai, Tahu, and John Taylor, eds. 2016. *Indigenous Data Sovereignty: Toward an Agenda*. Acton, ACT, Australia: Australian National University Press.

Lambek, Michael. 2010. *Ordinary Ethics: Anthropology, Language, and Action*. New York: Fordham University Press.

Lambert, Valerie. 2022. *Native Agency: Indians in the Bureau of Indian Affairs.* Indigenous Americas. Minneapolis: University of Minnesota Press.

Langwick, Stacey A. 2008. "Articulate(d) Bodies: Traditional Medicine in a Tanzanian Hospital." *American Ethnologist* 35 (3): 428–39. https://doi.org/10.1111/j.1548-1425.2008.00044.x.

———. 2011. *Bodies, Politics, and African Healing the Matter of Maladies in Tanzania.* Bloomington: Indiana University Press. http://site.ebrary.com/id/10481727.

———. 2018. "A Politics of Habitability: Plants, Healing, and Sovereignty in a Toxic World." *Cultural Anthropology* 33 (3): 415–43.

Lara, Ana-Maurine. 2020. *Queer Freedom: Black Sovereignty.* New York: SUNY Press.

Larme, Anne C., and Thomas L Leatherman. 2003. "Why Sobreparto? Women's Work, Health, and Reproduction in Two Districts in Southern Peru." In *Medical Pluralism in the Andes,* ed. Joan Koss-Chioino, Thomas L. Leatherman, and Christine Greenway, 211–28. Theory and Practice in Medical Anthropology and International Health. London; New York: Routledge.

Latour, Bruno. 1993. *We Have Never Been Modern.* Cambridge, MA: Harvard University Press.

———. 2004. "Why Has Critique Run Out of Steam? From Matters of Fact to Matters of Concern." *Critical Inquiry* 30 (2): 225–48. https://doi.org/10.1086/421123.

Laurens, Vivian, César Abadía-Barrero, and Mario Hernández. 2023. "Latin American Social Medicine in Colombia: Violence, Neoliberalism, and Buen Vivir." *The Journal of Latin American and Caribbean Anthropology* 28 (2): 93–105. https://doi.org/10.1111/jlca.12657.

Lawrence, David S., and Lioba A Hirsch. 2020. "Decolonising Global Health: Transnational Research Partnerships Under the Spotlight." *International Health* 12 (6): 518–23. https://doi.org/10.1093/inthealth/ihaa073.

Lazar, Sian. 2008. *El Alto, Rebel City: Self and Citizenship in Andean Bolivia.* Durham, NC: Duke University Press.

Lea, Tess. 2020. *Wild Policy.* Stanford, CA: Stanford University Press.

Ledo, Carmen, and René Soria. 2011. "Sistema de Salud de Bolivia." *Salud Pública de México* 53 (2).

Lehm Ardaya, Zulema, and Silvia Rivera Cusicanqui. 1988. *Los Artesanos Libertarios y La Ética Del Trabajo.* La Paz, Bolivia: Ediciones del THOA.

Leinaweaver, Jessaca. 2008. *The Circulation of Children: Kinship, Adoption, and Morality in Andean Peru.* Durham, NC, and London: Duke University Press.

Li, Tania. 2007. *The Will to Improve: Governmentality, Development, and the Practice of Politics.* Durham, NC: Duke University Press.

Liboiron, Max. 2021. *Pollution Is Colonialism.* Durham, NC: Duke University Press.

Livingston, Julie. 2012. *Improvising Medicine: An African Oncology Ward in an Emerging Cancer Epidemic.* Durham, NC: Duke University Press.

Locklear, Sofia, Martell Hesketh, Natalyn Begay, Jennifer Brixey, Abigail Echo-Hawk, and Rosalina James. 2023. "Reclaiming Our Narratives: An Indigenous Evaluation Framework for Urban American Indian/Alaska Native Communities." *Canadian Journal of Program Evaluation* 38 (1): 8–26. https://doi.org/10.3138/cjpe.75518.

Lowe, Lisa. 2015. *The Intimacies of Four Continents.* Durham, NC: Duke University Press.

Loza, Carmen Beatriz. 2008. *El Laberinto de La Curación: Itinerarios Terapéuticos En Las Ciudades de La Paz y El Alto.* La Paz, Bolivia: ISEAT.

———. 2013. "¿La Disminución de La Mortalidad Materna Es Un Simple Problema Técnico de Adecuación Cultural?" *História, Ciências, Saúde-Manguinhos* 20 (3): 1082–86.

Loza, Carmen Beatriz, and Walter Álvarez Quispe. 2011. *Sobreparto de La Mujer Indígena: Saberes y Prácticas Para Reducir La Muerte Materna.* La Paz, Bolivia: Instituto Boliviano de Medicina Tradicional Kallawaya.

Lugones, Maria. 2007. "Heterosexualism and the Colonial/Modern Gender System." *Hypatia* 22 (1): 186–219.

Maclean, Kate. 2023. *Cash, Clothes, and Construction: Rethinking Value in Bolivia's Pluri-Economy.* Minneapolis, University of Minnesota Press.

Macusaya Cruz, Carlos. 2014. *Desde El Sujeto Racializado:Consideraciones Sobre El Pensamiento Indianista de Fausto Reinaga.* La Paz, Bolivia: Minka.

———. 2020. *En Bolivia No Hay Racismo, Indios de Mierda: Apuntes Sobre Un Problema Negado.* La Paz, Bolivia: Edicioned Jiccha.

Maldonado-Torres, Nelson. 2007. "On the Coloniality of Being: Contributions to the Development of a Concept." *Cultural Studies* 21 (2–3): 240–70.

Mamani Ramirez, Pablo. 2004. "El Rugir de La Multitud: Levantamiento de La Ciudad Aymara de El Alto y Caída Del Gobierno de Sánchez de Lozada." *Temas Sociales* 25: 118–34.

Martínez, Rebecca G. 2018. *Marked Women: The Cultural Politics of Cervical Cancer in Venezuela.* Stanford, CA: Stanford University Press.

Mason, Katherine A. 2018. "Quantitative Care: Caring for the Aggregate in US Academic Population Health Sciences: Quantitative Care." *American Ethnologist* 45 (2): 201–13. https://doi.org/10.1111/amet.12632.

Matza, Tomas. 2018. *Shock Therapy: Psychology, Precarity, and Well-Being in Postsocialist Russia.* Durham, NC: Duke University Press.

Maurer, Megan. 2020. "Nourishing Environments, Caring Cities: Gardening and the Social Reproduction of the Urban Environment in Deindustrial Michigan." *City & Society* 32 (3): 716–37. https://doi.org/10.1111/ciso.12347.

McKay, Ramah. 2018. *Medicine in the Meantime: The Work of Care in Mozambique*. Durham, NC: Duke University Press.

McNelly, Angus. 2023. *Now We Are in Power: The Politics of Passive Revolution in Twenty-First Century Bolivia*. Pitt Latin American Series. Pittsburgh: University of Pittsburgh Press.

Medina, Javier. 2001. *Suma Qamaña : La Comprensión Indígena de La Buena Vida*. *Proyecto de Apoyo a La Gestión Participativa Municipal*. La Paz, Bolivia: Deutsche Gesellschaft für Technische Zusammenarbeit (GTZ); Federación de Asociaciones Municipales de Bolivia.

Meehan, Katie, and Kendra Stauss. 2015. *Precarious Worlds: Contested Geographies of Social Reproduction*. Athens: University of Georgia Press.

Mendizabal Lozano, Gregorio. 2002. *Historia de La Salud Pública En Bolivia: De Las Juntas de Sanidad a Los Directorios Locales de Salud*. La Paz, Bolivia: Prisa Ltda.

Mendoza, Breny. 2020. "Decolonial Theories in Comparison." *Journal of World Philosophies* 5 (1): 43–60.

Menéndez, Eduardo. 1992. "Modelo Hegemónico, Modelo Alternativo Subordinado, Modelo de Autoatención. Caracteres Estructurales." *La Antropología Médica En México*, 97–111.

Mignolo, Walter. 2010. "The Communal and the Decolonial." *Turbulence* 5. http://turbulence.org.uk/turbulence-5/decolonial/.

———. 2012. *Local Histories/Global Designs: Coloniality, Subaltern Knowledges, and Border Thinking*. Princeton, NJ: Princeton University Press.

Million, Dian. 2013. *Therapeutic Nations: Healing in an Age of Indigenous Human Rights*. Tucson: University of Arizona Press.

———. 2020. "Resurgent Kinships: Indigenous Relations of Well-Being vs. Humanitarian Health Economies." In *Routledge Handbook of Critical Indigenous Studies*, ed. Brendan Hokowhitu, Aileen Moreton-Robinson, Linda Tuhiwai-Smith, Chris Andersen, and Steve Larkin. Abingdon, Oxon, UK, and New York: Routledge.

Ministerio de Planificación del Desarollo. 2007. "Plan Nacional de Desarollo: 'Bolivia Digna, Soberana, Productiva y Democrática Para Vivir Bien.'"

Ministerio de Salud de Bolivia. 2014. *Curso de Educación Permanente En La Política de Salud Familiar Comunitaria Intercultural y El Sistema Único de Salud*. La Paz, Bolivia: Ministerio de Salud de Bolivia.

Ministerio de Salud y Deportes. 2006. *Protocolos de Atención Materna y Neonatal Culturalmente Adecuados*. La Paz, Bolivia: Ministerio de Salud y Deportes.

———. 2008. *Norma Nacional: Red Municipal de Salud Familiar Comunitaria Inter-*

cultural: Red Municipal SAFCI y Red de Servicios. La Paz, Bolivia: Ministerio de Salud y Deportes.

———. 2019. "Instructivo de Llenado: Carpeta Familiar." La Paz, Bolivia: Ministerio de Salud y Deportes.

Mintz, Sidney W., and Eric R. Wolf. 1950. "An Analysis of Ritual Co-Parenthood (Compadrazgo)." *Southwestern Journal of Anthropology* 6 (4): 341–68. https://doi.org/10.2307/3628562.

Mol, Annemarie. 2008. *The Logic of Care: Health and the Problem of Patient Choice*. New York: Routledge.

Mol, Annemarie, Ingunn Moser, and Jeannette Pols, eds. 2015. *Care in Practice: On Tinkering in Clinics, Homes and Farms*. Bielefeld, Germany: Transcript Publishing.

Molina, Fernando. 2021. *Racismo y Poder En Bolivia*. La Paz, Bolivia: Plural Editores.

Moraña, Mabel, Enrique D. Dussel, and Carlos A. Jáuregui. 2008. "Colonialism and Its Replicants." In *Coloniality at Large: Latin America and the Postcolonial Debate*, ed. Mabel Moraña, Enrique D. Dussel, and Carlos A. Jáuregui, 1–22. Durham, NC: Duke University Press.

Morgan, Lynn M. 1987. "Dependency Theory in the Political Economy of Health: An Anthropological Critique." *Medical Anthropology Quarterly* 1 (2): 131–54.

Morgensen, Scott Lauria. 2011. "The Biopolitics of Settler Colonialism: Right Here, Right Now." *Settler Colonial Studies* 1 (1): 52–76. https://doi.org/10.1080/2201473X.2011.10648801.

Mosse, David. 2004. "Is Good Policy Unimplementable? Reflections on the Ethnography of Aid Policy and Practice." *Development and Change* 35 (4): 639–71.

———. 2005. *Cultivating Development: An Ethnography of Aid Policy and Practice*. London: Pluto Press.

Murphy, Michelle. 2015. "Unsettling Care: Troubling Transnational Itineraries of Care in Feminist Health Practices." *Social Studies of Science* 45 (5): 717–37.

Nash, June. 1993. *We Eat the Mines and the Mines Eat Us: Dependency and Exploitation in Bolivian Mines*. New York: Columbia University Press.

Navaro-Yashin, Yael. 2002. *Faces of the State: Secularism and Public Life in Turkey*. Princeton, NJ: Princeton University Press.

Ngai, Sianne. 2005. *Ugly Feelings*. Cambridge, MA: Harvard University Press.

Nguyen, Vinh-Kim. 2010. *The Republic of Therapy: Triage and Sovereignty in West Africa's Time of AIDS*. Durham, NC: Duke University Press.

Nigenda, Gustavo, Gerardo Mora-Flores, Salvador Aldama-López, and Emanuel Orozco-Núñez. 2001. "La Práctica de La Medicina Tradicional En

América Latina y El Caribe: El Dilema Entre Regulación y Tolerancia." *Salud Pública Mexico* 43 (1): 41–51. https://doi.org/10.1590/S0036-363420010 00100006.

Ong, Aihwa. 2010. *Spirits of Resistance and Capitalist Discipline: Factory Women in Malaysia.* 2nd ed. SUNY Series in the Anthropology of Work. Albany, NY: SUNY Press.

Orta, Andrew. 2004. *Catechizing Culture: Missionaries, Aymara, and the "New Evangelization."* New York: Columbia University Press. https://doi.org/10.73 12/orta13068.

Pachaguaya Yujra, Pedro, and Claudia Terrazas Sosa. 2020. *Una Cuarentena Individual Para Una Sociedad Colectiva: La Llegada y Despacho Del Khapaj Niño Coronavirus a Bolivia.* La Paz, Bolivia: Asociación Departamental de Antropólogos de La Paz.

Pacino, Nicole. 2013. "Constructing a New Bolivian Society: Public Health Reforms and the Consolidation of the Bolivian National Revolution." *The Latin Americanist,* 25–55.

———. 2015. "Creating Madres Campesinas: Revolutionary Motherhood and the Gendered Politics of Nation Building in 1950s Bolivia." *Journal of Women's History* 27 (1): 62–87.

Palmié, Stephan. 2002. *Wizards and Scientists: Explorations in Afro-Cuban Modernity and Tradition.* Durham, NC, and London: Duke University Press.

Patzi Paco, Félix. 2004. *Sistema Comunal: Una Propuesta Alternativa al Sistema Liberal.* La Paz, Bolivia: Comunidad de Estudios Alternativos.

———. 2014. *Miseria de La Ley Avelino Siñani y Elizardo Pérez En Su Fase de Implementación.* La Paz, Bolivia: Editorial Vicuña.

Pérez-Bustos, Tania. 2017. "A Word of Caution Toward Homogenous Appropriations of Decolonial Thinking in STS." *Catalyst: Feminism, Theory, Technoscience* 3 (1).

Pigg, Stacy Leigh. 1996. "The Credible and the Credulous: The Question of 'Villagers' Beliefs' in Nepal." *Cultural Anthropology* 11 (2): 160–201.

———. 1997. "'Found in Most Traditional Societies': Traditional Medical Practitioners Between Culture and Development." In *International Development and the Social Sciences: Essays on the History and Politics of Knowledge,* ed. Frederick Cooper and Randall M. Packard, 259–90. Berkeley: University of California Press. http://search.ebscohost.com/login.aspx?direct=true&scope=site&db=nlebk&db=nlabk&AN=41865.

Pigg, Stacy Leigh, Susan L. Erikson, and Kathleen Inglis. 2018. "Introduction: Document/Ation: Power, Interests, Accountabilities." *Anthropologica* 60 (1): 167–77.

Pinto, Sarah. 2008. *Where There Is No Midwife: Birth and Loss in Rural India.* New York: Berghahn Books.

Platt, Tristan. 2013. "Care and Carelessness in Rural Bolivia. Silence and Emotion in Quechua Childbirth Testimonies." *Bulletin de l'Institut Français d'études Andines* 42 (3): 333–51. https://doi.org/10.4000/bifea.4113.

Pols, Jeannette, and Ingunn Moser. 2009. "Cold Technologies Versus Warm Care? On Affective and Social Relations with and Through Care Technologies." *Alter* 3 (2): 159–78.

Portugal Mollinedo, Pedro. 2011. "Visión Posmoderna y Visión Andina Del Desarollo." In *El Desarollo En Questión: Reflexiones Desde América Latina*, ed. Fernanda Wanderley, 253–82. La Paz, Bolivia: CIDES-UMSA.

Postero, Nancy. 2007. *Now We Are Citizens: Indigenous Politics in Postmulticultural Bolivia*. Stanford, CA: Stanford University Press.

—— 2017. *The Indigenous State: Race, Politics, and Performance in Plurinational Bolivia*. Oakland: University of California Press.

Povinelli, Elizabeth A. 2002. *The Cunning of Recognition: Indigenous Alterities and the Making of Australian Multiculturalism*. Durham, NC: Duke University Press.

Praspaliauskiene, Rima. 2016. "Enveloped Lives: Practicing Health and Care in Lithuania." *Medical Anthropology Quarterly* 30 (4): 582–98. https://doi.org/10.1111/maq.12291.

Puig de la Bellacasa, Maria. 2017. *Matters of Care: Speculative Ethics in More Than Human Worlds*. Minneapolis: University of Minnesota Press.

Quijano, Aníbal. 1999. "Colonialidad Del Poder, Cultura y Conocimiento En América Latina." *Dispositio* 24 (41): 137–48.

——. 2000. "Coloniality of Power and Eurocentrism in Latin America." *International Sociology* 15 (2): 215–32.

Ramírez Hita, Susana. 2008. "Políticas de Salud Basadas En El Concepto de Interculturalidad. Los Centros de Salud Intercultural En El Altiplano Boliviano." *IX Congreso Argentino de Antropología Social*.

Ramones, Ikaika, and Sally Engle Merry. 2021. "Capitalist Transformation and Settler Colonialism: Theorizing the Interface." *American Anthropologist* 123 (4): 741–52. https://doi.org/10.1111/aman.13655.

Randle, Sayd. 2022. "Ecosystem Duties, Green Infrastructure, and Environmental Injustice in Los Angeles." *American Anthropologist* 124 (1): 77–89. https://doi.org/10.1111/aman.13650.

Rappaport, Joanne. 2005. *Intercultural Utopias: Public Intellectuals, Cultural Experimentation, and Ethnic Pluralism in Colombia*. Durham, NC: Duke University Press.

Ravindran, Tathagatan. 2020. "What Undecidability Does: Enduring Racism in the Context of Indigenous Resurgence in Bolivia." *Ethnic and Racial Studies* 43 (6): 976–94. https://doi.org/10.1080/01419870.2019.1628997.

——. 2021. "The Power of Phenotype: Toward an Ethnography of Pigmentocracy in Andean Bolivia." *The Journal of Latin American and Caribbean Anthropology* 26 (2): 219–36. https://doi.org/10.1111/jlca.12551.

Reese, Ashanté M. 2019. *Black Food Geographies: Race, Self-Reliance, and Food Access in Washington, D.C.* Chapel Hill: University of North Carolina Press.

Regalsky, Pablo. 2005. *Territorio e Interculturalidad: La Participación Campesina Indígena y La Reconfiguración Del Espacio Andino Rural.* La Paz, Bolivia: Editora Proeib Andes.

———. 2009. *Las Paradojas Del Proceso Constituyente Boliviano.* Centro de Comunicación y Desarrolllo Andino, CENDA.

———. 2010. "Political Processes and the Reconfiguration of the State in Bolivia." *Latin American Perspectives* 37 (3): 35–50.

Reinaga, Fausto. 1940. *Mitayos Y Yanaconas.* Oruro, Bolivia: Imprenta Mazuelo Oruro.

———. 1969. *La Revolución India.* 1. La Paz: Ediciones PIB (Partido Indio de Bolivia).

Richardson, Eugene T. 2020. *Epidemic Illusions: On the Coloniality of Global Public Health.* Cambridge, MA: MIT Press.

Riofrancos, Thea. 2020. *Resource Radicals: From Petro-Nationalism to Post-Extractivism in Ecuador.* Durham, NC: Duke University Press.

Rivera Cusicanqui, Silvia. 1984. *Oprimidos Pero No Vencidos: Luchas Del Campesinado Aymara y Qhechwa de Bolivia, 1900–1980. Serie Movimientos Sociales.* La Paz, Bolivia: HISBOL: CSUTCB.

———. 1990. "Liberal Democracy and Ayllu Democracy in Bolivia: The Case of Northern Potosí." Trans. Charles Roberts. *Journal of Development Studies* 26 (4): 97–121. https://doi.org/10.1080/00220389008422175.

———. 1991. *Pachakuti: Los Aymara de Bolivia Frente a Medio Milenio de Colonialismo. Serie Cuadernos de Debate.* Chukiyawu La Paz, Bolivia: Taller de Historia Oral Andina.

———. 2010. *Violencias (Re) Encubiertas.* La Paz, Bolivia: Editorial Piedra Rota.

———. 2014. *Mito y Desarrollo En Bolivia: El Giro Colonial Del Gobierno Del MAS.* La Paz, Bolivia: Plural Editores.

Robbins, Joel. 2009. "Value, Structure, and the Range of Possibilities: A Response to Zigon." *Ethnos,* 277–85.

Roberts, Elizabeth. 2012. *God's Laboratory: Assisted Reproduction in the Andes.* Berkeley, CA: University of California Press.

Rosa, Jonathan. 2019. *Looking Like a Language, Sounding Like a Race: Raciolinguistic Ideologies and the Learning of Latinidad.* Oxford Studies in the Anthropology of Language. New York: Oxford University Press.

Salas Carreño, Guillermo. 2019. "Evangelicalism in the Rural Andes." In *The Andean World,* ed. Linda J. Seligmann, 280–96. The Routledge Worlds. New York: Routledge.

Salazar, Huáscar. 2020. "Bolivia: la necesidad de invertir en la salud de la po-blación." El País Tarija. November 30, 2020. https://elpais.bo/reportajes/20 201130_bolivia-la-necesidad-de-invertir-en-la-salud-de-la-poblacion.html.

Saldaña-Portillo, María. 2016. *Indian Given: Racial Geographies Across Mexico and the United States*. Durham, NC, and London: Duke University Press.

Saluk, Seda. 2022. "Datafied Pregnancies: Health Information Technologies and Reproductive Governance in Turkey." *Medical Anthropology Quarterly* 36 (1): 101–18. https://doi.org/10.1111/maq.12675.

Salzinger, Leslie. 2003. *Genders in Production: Making Workers in Mexico's Global Factories*. Berkeley: University of California Press.

Sanabria, Emilia. 2016. *Plastic Bodies: Sex Hormones and Menstrual Suppression in Brazil*. Durham, NC, and London: Duke University Press.

Sanjinés, Javier. 2004. *Mestizaje Upside-Down: Aesthetic Politics in Modern Bo-livia*. Pittsburgh: University of Pittsburgh Press.

Schavelzón, Salvador. 2012. "El Nacimiento Del Estado Plurinacional de Bo-livia: Etnografía de Una Asamblea Constituyente." Federal University of Rio de Janeiro.

Scherz, China. 2011. "Protecting Children, Preserving Families: Moral Con-flict and Actuarial Science in a Problem of Contemporary Governance." *PoLAR: Political and Legal Anthropology Review* 34 (1): 33–50. https://doi.org/10.1111/j.1555-2934.2011.01137.x.

———. 2014. *Having People, Having Heart: Charity, Sustainable Development, and Problems of Dependence in Central Uganda*. Chicago; London: University of Chicago Press.

Schiller, Naomi. 2018. *Channeling the State: Community Media and Popular Politics in Venezuela*. Radical Américas. Durham, NC: Duke University Press.

Scott, James C. 1998. *Seeing Like a State: How Certain Schemes to Improve the Human Condition Have Failed*. New Haven, CT: Yale University Press.

Segato, Rita Laura. 2013. *La Crítica de La Colonialidad En Ocho Ensayos: Y Una Antropología Por Demanda*. n.c.: Prometeo libros.

———. 2016. "Patriarchy from Margin to Center: Discipline, Territoriality, and Cruelty in the Apocalyptic Phase of Capital." *South Atlantic Quarterly* 115 (3): 615–24. https://doi.org/10.1215/00382876-3608675.

Shakow, Miriam. 2011. "The Peril and Promise of Noodles and Beer: Condem-nation of Patronage and Hybrid Political Frameworks in 'Post-Neoliberal' Cochabamba, Bolivia." *PoLAR: Political and Legal Anthropology Review* 34 (2): 315–36. https://doi.org/10.1111/j.1555-2934.2011.01168.x.

———. 2014. *Along the Bolivian Highway: Social Mobility and Political Culture in a New Middle Class*. Contemporary Ethnography. Philadelphia: University of Pennsylvania Press.

Shange, Savannah. 2019. *Progressive Dystopia: Abolition, Antiblackness, and Schooling in San Francisco*. Durham, NC: Duke University Press.

Sheehan, Helen. 2009. "Medical Pluralism in India: Patient Choice or No Other Options?" *Indian Journal of Medical Ethics* 6: 138–41.

Siekmeier, James F. 2011. *The Bolivian Revolution and the United States, 1952 to the Present*. University Park, PA: Pennsylvania State University Press.

Sikkink, Lynn. 2010. *New Cures, Old Medicines: Women and the Commercialization of Traditional Medicine in Bolivia*. Case Studies in Cultural Anthropology. Belmont, CA: Wadsworth.

Simpson, Audra. 2014. *Mohawk Interruptus: Political Life Across the Borders of Settler States*. Durham, NC: Duke University Press.

———. 2016. "The State Is a Man: Theresa Spence, Loretta Saunders and the Gender of Settler Sovereignty." *Theory & Event* 19 (4).

———. 2020. "Empire of Feeling." *Bulletin of the General Anthropology Division* 27 (1): 1–8.

Singer, Elyse Ona. 2022. *Lawful Sins: Abortion Rights and Reproductive Governance in Mexico*. Stanford, CA: Stanford University Press.

Spedding, Alison. 1997. "The Coca Field as a Total Social Fact." In *Coca, Cocaine, and the Bolivian Reality*, ed. Madeline Barbara Léons and Harry Sanabria, 47–70. Albany, NY: SUNY Press.

Speed, Shannon. 2017. "Structures of Settler Capitalism in Abya Yala." *American Quarterly* 69 (4): 783–90.

Stepan, Nancy. 1991. *The Hour of Eugenics: Race, Gender, and Nation in Latin America*. Ithaca, NY: Cornell University Press.

Stevenson, Lisa. 2014. *Life Beside Itself: Imagining Care in the Canadian Arctic*. Oakland: University of California Press.

Stoler, Ann Laura. 1995. *Race and the Education of Desire: Foucault's History of Sexuality and the Colonial Order of Things*. Durham, NC: Duke University Press.

———. 2010. *Carnal Knowledge and Imperial Power: Race and the Intimate in Colonial Rule: With a New Preface*. Berkeley: University of California Press.

Strathern, Marilyn. 2005. *Kinship, Law and the Unexpected: Relatives Are Always a Surprise*. 1st ed. Cambridge, UK: Cambridge University Press.

Street, Alice. 2014. *Biomedicine in an Unstable Place: Intrastructure and Personhood in a Papua New Guinea Hospital*. Durham, NC: Duke University Press.

Strong, Adrienne E. 2020. *Documenting Death: Maternal Mortality and the Ethics of Care in Tanzania*. Oakland: University of California Press.

Stuelke, Patricia. 2021. *The Ruse of Repair: US Neoliberal Empire and the Turn from Critique*. Durham, NC: Duke University Press.

Suh, Siri. 2021. *Dying to Count: Post-Abortion Care and Global Reproductive Health Politics in Senegal*. Medical Anthropology. New Brunswick, NJ: Rutgers University Press.

Táíwò, Olúfẹ́mi O. 2022. *Elite Capture: How the Powerful Took Over Identity Politics (and Everything Else)*. Chicago: Haymarket Books.

TallBear, Kim. 2013. *Native American DNA*. Minneapolis: University of Minnesota Press.

———. 2017. "Beyond the Life/Not Life Binary: A Feminist-Indigenous Reading of Cryopreservation, Interspecies Thinking and the New Materialisms." In *Cryopolitics*, 179–202.

———. 2019. "Caretaking Relations, Not American Dreaming." *Kalfou* 6 (1).

Tapias, Maria. 2015. *Embodied Protests: Emotions and Women's Health in Bolivia*. Champaign: University of Illinois Press.

Tassi, Nico. 2010. "The 'Postulate of Abundance': Cholo Market and Religion in La Paz, Bolivia." *Social Anthropology* 18 (2): 191–209.

———. 2017. *The Native World-System: An Ethnography of Bolivian Aymara Traders in the Global Economy*. Issues of Globalization: Case Studies in Contemporary Anthropology. New York; Oxford, UK: Oxford University Press.

Taussig, Michael. 2010. *The Devil and Commodity Fetishism in South America*. 30th ed. Chapel Hill: University of North Carolina Press.

Ticktin, Miriam. 2011. *Casualties of Care: Immigration and the Politics of Humanitarianism in France*. Berkeley: University of California Press.

Todd, Zoe. 2015. "Indigenizing the Anthropocene." In *Art in the Anthropocene: Encounters among Aesthetics, Politics, Environments and Epistemologies*, ed. Heather Davis and Etienne Turpin, 241–54. Critical Climate Change. London: Open Humanities Press.

———. 2016. "An Indigenous Feminist's Take on the Ontological Turn: 'Ontology' Is Just Another Word for Colonialism." *Journal of Historical Sociology* 29 (1): 4–22.

———. 2018. "Refracting the State Through Human-Fish Relations: Fishing, Indigenous Legal Orders and Colonialism in North/Western Canada." *Decolonization: Indigeneity, Education & Society* 7 (1): 60–75.

Torres-Goita, Javier. 2010. "Movilización Popular Por La Salud En Bolivia." *Estudios Sobre La Culturas Contemporaneas* 16 (31).

Torres Goitia, Javier, and Mario Burgoa. 2015. *La Salud Como Derecho: Conquista y Evolución En Bolivia*. La Paz, Bolivia: Plural Editores.

Tórrez Eguino, Mario. 2012. *Suma Qamaña y Desarollo: El t'hinkhu Necesario*. Cooperación Suiza en Bolivia (COSUDE).

Trigo, María Silvia, Anatoly Kurmanaev, and Allison McCann. 2020. "As Politicians Clashed, Bolivia's Pandemic Death Rate Soared." *New York Times*, August 22, 2020, sec. World. https://www.nytimes.com/2020/08/22/world/americas/virus-bolivia.html.

Tsing, Anna Lowenhaupt. 2015. *The Mushroom at the End of the World: On the Possibility of Life in Capitalist Ruins*. Princeton, NJ: Princeton University Press. https://doi.org/10.1515/9781400873548.

Tuck, Eve. 2009. "Suspending Damage: A Letter to Communities." *Harvard Educational Review* 79 (3): 409–28. https://doi.org/10.17763/haer.79.3.n00166 75661t3n15.

———. 2016. "Red and Black DNA, Blood, Kinship and Organizing." The Henceforward. http://www.thehenceforward.com/episodes/2016/7/25/episode-3 -red-and-black-dna-blood-kinship-and-organizing-with-kim-tallbear (accessed July 25, 2016).

Tuck, Eve, and K. Wayne Yang. 2012. "Decolonization Is Not a Metaphor." *Decolonization: Indigeneity, Education, & Society* 1 (1): 1–40.

United Nations Population Fund (UNFPA). 2012. *Las Compañeras En El Alumbrar. Dejando La Penumbra En El Arte Obstétrico. Bolivia, 1837–2012.* La Paz, Bolivia: United Nations Population Fund (UNFPA).

Valdivia Rivera, Soledad. 2021. "Introduction: Continuity and Change in the 2019–2020 Bolivian Crisis." In *Bolivia at the Crossroads: Politics, Economy, and Environment in a Time of Crisis,* ed. Soledad Valdivia Rivera. 1st ed. Abingdon, Oxon; New York: Routledge. Routledge. https://doi.org/10.4324 /9781003147923.

Van Vleet, Krista E. 2008. *Performing Kinship: Narrative, Gender, and the Intimacies of Power in the Andes.* 1st ed. Austin: University of Texas Press.

———. 2011. "On Devils and the Dissolution of Sociality: Andean Catholics Voicing Ambivalence in Neoliberal Bolivia." *Anthropological Quarterly* 84 (4): 835–64.

———. 2019. *Hierarchies of Care: Girls, Motherhood, and Inequality in Peru.* Champaign: University of Illinois Press.

Vargas, Yolanda. 2013. "Salud Familiar Comunitaria Intercultural (SAFCI)." In *Salud Materna En Contextos de Interculturalidad: Estudio de Los Pueblos Aymara, Ayoreode, Chiquitano, Guaraní, Quechua y Yuqui,* ed. Manigeh Roosta G., Primera edición, 35–72. La Paz, Bolivia: CIDES-UMSA.

Vega, Rosalynn. 2018. *No Alternative: Childbirth, Citizenship, and Indigenous Culture in Mexico.* Austin: University of Texas Press.

Velasco Guachalla, V. Ximena, Calla Hummel, Jami Nelson-Nuñez, and Carew Boulding. 2021. "Compounding Crises: Bolivia in 2020." *Revista de Ciencia Política (Santiago)* 41 (2): 211–37. https://doi.org/10.4067/S0718-090X202100 5000116.

Vogel, Lise. 2013. *Marxism and the Oppression of Women: Toward a Unitary Theory.* Leiden, Netherlands: Brill.

Wade, Peter. 2010. *Race and Ethnicity in Latin America.* 2nd ed. London; New York: Pluto Press; distributed in the United States of America exclusively by Palgrave Macmillan.

Waitzkin, Howard, Celia Iriart, Alfredo Estrada, and Silvia Lamadrid. 2001.

The authorized representative in the EU for product safety and compliance is:
Mare Nostrum Group B.V.
Mauritskade 21D
1091 GC Amsterdam
The Netherlands
Email address: gpsr@mare-nostrum.co.uk

KVK chamber of commerce number: 96249943